GORDON SHARP

GOING
FOR A
SPIN

THE UPS AND DOWNS OF AN AEROSPACE DOCTOR

GORDON SHARP

GOING FOR A SPIN

THE UPS AND DOWNS OF AN AEROSPACE DOCTOR

MEREO
Cirencester

Mereo Books

1A The Wool Market Dyer Street Cirencester Gloucestershire GL7 2PR
An imprint of Memoirs Publishing www.mereobooks.com

Going for a spin: 978-1-86151-214-7

First published in Great Britain in 2014
by Mereo Books, an imprint of Memoirs Publishing

Copyright ©2014

Gordon Sharp has asserted his right under the Copyright Designs and Patents Act 1988 to be identified as the author of this work.

A CIP catalogue record for this book is available from the British Library.

This book is sold subject to the condition that it shall not by way of trade or otherwise be lent, resold, hired out or otherwise circulated without the publisher's prior consent in any form of binding or cover, other than that in which it is published and without a similar condition, including this condition being imposed on the subsequent purchaser.

The address for Memoirs Publishing Group Limited can be found at
www.memoirspublishing.com

The Memoirs Publishing Group Ltd Reg. No. 7834348

The Memoirs Publishing Group supports both The Forest Stewardship Council® (FSC®) and the PEFC® leading international forest-certification organisations. Our books carrying both the FSC label and the PEFC® and are printed on FSC®-certified paper. FSC® is the only forest-certification scheme supported by the leading environmental organisations including Greenpeace. Our paper procurement policy can be found at
www.memoirspublishing.com/environment

Cover design - Ray Lipscombe

Typeset in 10.5/15pt Plantin
by Wiltshire Associates Publisher Services Ltd. Printed and bound in Great Britain by Printondemand-Worldwide, Peterborough PE2 6XD

Contents

Foreword

Acknowledgements

Chapter 1	Bombers over Glasgow	P. 1
Chapter 2	An enquiring mind	P. 12
Chapter 3	Mr McCabe and the tree of life	P. 30
Chapter 4	Chamber and centrifuge	P. 59
Chapter 5	Desert boots and flying suits	P. 82
Chapter 6	A change in the wind	P. 113
Chapter 7	Spreading my wings	P. 138
Chapter 8	On air, and back down to earth	P. 160
Chapter 9	By Royal Appointment	P. 187
Chapter 10	Driving for a healthy workforce	P. 209
	Epilogue	P. 229

FOREWORD

This life is such a mad rush that it is only when we reach retirement age and can award ourselves a little time to sit back and think that we can reflect on all that has happened to us, and wonder what we might have done differently. Decisions which seemed trivial at the time, twists of fate which went unregarded, make all the difference; and so it was with me.

I have been lucky enough to enjoy a life which has perhaps brought me more than my share of adventure and achievement, despite a few of those inevitable frustrations, disappointments and occasional terrible heartaches we all have to endure. It has given me a fund of stories with which to amuse my children. It has also given me a first-hand glimpse, from time to time, of history in the making, and brought me into contact with some of the people who were making it; they include some remarkable, inspirational individuals who in many cases, to my great good fortune, became my friends.

While my memory is still clear, I have decided to commit my story to paper. If it helps to encourage even one individual from a younger generation to pursue a career in aviation medicine, I will consider it worthwhile. At the very least, I hope it will provide a little entertainment.

Gordon Sharp
Fortrose, March 2014

ACKNOWLEDGEMENTS

I should like to thank my old friend Arthur Ferns, his wife Marion and his family for their loyalty, friendship and great support over so many years. My thanks also to Chris Newton of Memoirs Books for his patient unravelling of a wealth of information to produce an account which is far more coherent than I could have managed alone, and to Ray Lipscombe for his superb design. And of course, my deepest love and thanks always to my dear wife Kirstie.

To my late son William
A great inspiration to us all.

CHAPTER ONE

BOMBERS OVER GLASGOW

I was not quite six years old when I decided I wanted to be a doctor, and it came about in the most cataclysmic and distressing manner.

I was living with my father and mother in our house in the west end of Glasgow; the year was 1941 and the date was March 13. That date will be inscribed upon my memory forever.

I was sound asleep in my bed on that Thursday evening when around nine o'clock, I was awoken by my mother, who gently told me that the air-raid siren had sounded and a bombing raid had just begun. We had been aware that this was a possibility because the extensive shipyards of Clydebank, just ten miles to the west of the city, were an obvious target for the Germans.

My mother assured me that I should not worry too much because the bombers would be targeting the Clyde shipyards and military installations further to the west. 'We should all be safe here' Mum said, although we wasted no time in seeking safety in our Morrison table shelter, which had been assembled in a downstairs spare bedroom. The Morrison shelter was like a giant cage with a heavy thick steel table top, designed for use indoors and intended to protect you from falling masonry if your house was hit and the floors collapsed. Mum quickly dressed me in my 'siren suit' over my pyjamas, a cosy one-piece garment which Mum had sewn up for me to a design similar to the one Mr Churchill had made for use at night in the cold underground War Cabinet rooms during the London Blitz, and the three of us squeezed into the Morrison shelter. I could tell my parents were worried, although they disguised it well, and although I was a little alarmed, I believed their assurances that we would all be safe. In fact, I found the situation quite exciting and wanted to look out the window to see the aeroplanes going over the house. The bombing continued however, and the whistle of falling bombs and the 'crump' as they found their target seemed to get more intensive. I slept the sleep of the innocent, quite unaware of the drama that was building up in the skies above Clydebank.

Some time after midnight I was awoken again, to be told that we were going to have to leave the house and move into the greater safety of the outdoor Anderson shelter in the garden. I knew that Anderson shelter well. I had watched the workmen dig a deep hole at the bottom of our garden, roof it over with corrugated iron plates and cover the whole thing with sandbags and earth. I had been told not to play in the shelter, but my friend and neighbour Bertie and I frequently used it as a play 'submarine', so the damp, dank smell of what was to be our 'bedroom' that night was quite familiar to me.

When my mother led me outside it seemed very bright, almost like day. There was a full moon, and the air was filled with the throbbing of German bombers, a sinister, pulsating roar; we could hear the rattle of the anti-aircraft guns trying to bring them down (we learned later that they had had little if any success). We could see a red glow coming from Clydebank, which was about ten or twelve miles away to the west. There was a smell of burning, and as we walked down the garden there came a sudden flash as a bomb exploded nearby.

My father had gone out on patrol with an ARP warden, but suddenly he appeared at the shelter door. He said a parachutist had been spotted coming down in the field behind our house, and he had come to collect his axe and tools so he could deal with him. If only it had been just a parachutist, but it wasn't – it was a land mine, and the wind was carrying it towards a group of houses nearby.

The next thing I knew was the most unspeakably loud noise - it sounded like the roar of an express train - followed by a loud 'whoosh'. The ground beneath us started to shake violently and debris and choking dust rained down on us. I was lifted clean out of my chair by the blast and knocked unconscious. When I came to I saw that my mother had been blown clear across the room, though mercifully she was not badly hurt.

Naturally, her first concern was for me, and she was clearly relieved to find that I was still alive. There I was sitting on the floor of the shelter surrounded by debris and covered in dust and blood – it was my blood, for there was a great gash in my right leg.

It soon emerged that by comparison with our neighbours,

we had had a lucky escape. Many of the houses around us, those which had taken the full force of the landmine, had either vanished or been reduced to piles of smoking rubble. It seemed that although we in the Kelvindale area of the City had not been the target of the bombers, we were unfortunate enough to lie under their return flight path, and one of them (probably to reduce weight for the return flight) had decided to despatch its left-over bombs as it passed overhead.

The raids of that night and the one that followed were among the most devastating of the Second World War. When the Germans were done with their death and destruction, over 500 people had died and many more lay seriously injured. Of approximately 12,000 houses in Clydebank itself, only seven remained undamaged. 4,000 had been completely destroyed and 4,500 severely damaged.

In his book *Luftwaffe over Scotland: a history of German air attacks on Scotland, 1939-45*, Les Taylor, an amateur historian, called the Clydebank Blitz the most cataclysmic event wartime Scotland had to endure. He wrote that while the raid on 13 March was not intended as a terror attack, the one the following night was. However, he believed that although the blitz had been intended to crack morale, it had had quite the opposite effect, strengthening resolve for the conflict among Scottish people. The Germans had underestimated the courage and resilience of the Scots as they had the English. In fact the Clydebank blitz was not fully reported at the time, to avoid upsetting the population and damaging morale.

At least my parents were unhurt. Dad returned to the shelter, also covered in dust but greatly relieved that Mum and I were still in one piece. He described how when he had realised the 'German parachutist' was a land-mine he had tried to fling himself to the ground, but the blast of the detonating bomb kept him floating for what seemed ages. He was fortunately unhurt by his experience.

On his return to the shelter he had a quick look at my leg wound, then carried me in his arms up to a hastily-created casualty clearing station in a church hall at the end of the lane behind our house. I can still recall the scene I saw through the open doors of the hall. It was one of chaos, with the hall full of injured and possibly dying people. An ARP warden was there, and when he spotted me he told Dad that the sights were appalling and must not be witnessed by a young boy. He insisted that we should go no further than the tiny entrance hall, and it was there that an elderly doctor dressed my leg, using dressings and bandages which he extracted from an old Gladstone bag. Naturally I was terrified and in considerable pain (especially when he applied iodine to the wound), but his gentle tone and the way he dealt with me were so unperturbed, so reassuring. I had not had much contact with doctors before, and I was deeply impressed by this man and his calm air of expertise.

By now there seemed to be a lull in the bombing, although in the clear moonlight we could see smoke and flames reaching skywards. Dad decided that we should see the rest of the night out at the old family house, Monkland, a couple of miles or so east in the Hyndland district of Glasgow. Although Grandfather had died three years previously, Grandmother and my aunt had stayed on in the old house and Dad was naturally anxious to know if they were safe.

Before we set off in the early hours of the morning my parents made a rapid survey of the bomb damage to our own house. The roof had been blasted off, and it was now clearly fit only for partial demolition; it would probably need substantial rebuilding. Although roofless, the walls of the garage and my father's old Wolseley car inside it were intact. He got it going and literally bulldozed it through the rubble to get it out into the road.

We set off, but progress was extremely slow because of the rubble from the bombing and the crowds of people wandering through the streets, shocked, homeless, injured, bereaved, or indeed all four. It was a vision from hell. My mother clasped her hands over my eyes to protect me from the horrors, but I could not resist peeping through her fingers. I saw what I knew were dead bodies, bits of bodies and horribly injured people sobbing in pain and distress. Many of the dead were unclothed; it was a mystery to me then, but I later learned that this is one of the effects of bomb blast.

Among the crowds of sobbing, injured people, huddled figures were moving, doing their best to administer first aid and comfort. They were doctors, I suppose, and nurses, wardens and lay people with first-aid knowledge. My heart surged in pride and admiration at what those people were doing so selflessly, and how they comforted and healed even as the victims lay there in the dust and the blood.

That was when I knew that one day, I should like to join them. When I grew up, I decided quietly to myself, I was going to be a doctor, like the kind gentleman who had sorted me out in the casualty station. I never knew his name.

Before we started out we had heard that another stray bomb had fallen to the east of our house, but little did we know that the house it had struck was next door to the old family house, Monkland; it seemed as if the Germans had scored a right and left on the Sharp family. We arrived to find that the house wasn't there any more, or at least not much of it. There was nothing left but a wall and a chimney and a still smouldering pile of rubble. We had been dealt a double blow. At least my grandmother and aunt were safe and by some miracle had survived. When the siren went, they had taken refuge in a cellar and the collapsing house had absorbed most of the energy from the landmine. Although Grandmother had a surface head injury, the ARP warden and some soldiers had managed to extricate her and my aunt through a tunnel they had made in the rubble blocking the entrance to the cellar. A policeman on duty at the end of Turnberry Road told Dad that they had carried Grandma on an old door as a makeshift stretcher and she and my aunt had been taken to the home of another uncle and aunt in Kingsborough Gardens, a few hundred yards away and untouched by the bombing. That night we too found refuge in the billiard room of that house, and I managed to snatch some fitful sleep for what remained of the night.

As dawn broke the next morning, my parents and I drove back to Kelvindale in the old and trusted Wolseley to see what could be salvaged from our bombed-out home. There was the most appalling scene of devastation and still that lingering horrible pungent smell, a mixture of cordite explosive and brick or stone rubble. Dad picked his way carefully through fallen rafters and roof tiles and managed to get into the house. All our furniture and possessions, he told me, were covered in slivers of broken glass from the windows which had been blown in when the bomb struck. I was so relieved when Dad came out to the car clutching my two favourite possessions- my teddy bear and best of all, a Meccano model of a De Havilland Rapide biplane which my older cousin had given me when he left for boarding school. That aeroplane was especially precious, and it didn't have a scratch on it. I remember thinking, 'This is one aeroplane the Germans are not going to destroy'.

We were all glad to drive away from the scene, though saddened by what had happened to our happy home. Poor Mum was in tears as she tried to salvage what she could to let us start our lives over again.

Even more distressing were the sights that greeted us later that morning when we went round again to see if anything could be rescued from the old family home now that it was daylight. There was nothing left to salvage. That was perhaps one of the most distressing sights I have ever experienced. That old Victorian house was where my father had grown up, and we looked on it as our second home. I loved everything about it and adored the garden which I played in and explored. Happy days had been shattered for ever by the events of the last few hours.

As I looked at the ruins, I recalled how years before Mum had taken me after school to visit my grandfather at the 'big house' regularly, and I remembered often being asked by Grandpa to sing a song called 'Ma Ain Wee Hoose'. It was his favourite and if I made a good job of singing it, he would send me down to the cook to collect a chocolate biscuit, or if my rendering had been particularly to his liking I was rewarded with a slice of fruitcake. Other rewards were boiled sweets, toffees and chocolates, usually samples from one of Grandpa's three or four sweet factories. They were always available, and my aunt would dish them out in liberal quantities, much to Mum's concern, because of the likely damage to my teeth.

If I was stubborn and moodily refused to sing to Grandpa, I would be treated that evening to a dose of Gregory's Mixture, a foul-tasting laxative concoction which Mum believed was a cure-all for every mood change. Her faith in the dreaded mixture extended into the war years. At the outbreak of war, while everybody else stockpiled foodstuffs and other essentials, it seemed to me that Mum bought in enough Gregory's Mixture to give a regiment a 'good run for their money'. I loathed the foul taste and indeed, the laxative effects of the stuff, and I am sure the threat of a bedtime dose kept my singing voice well up to scratch. The latter was not one of the happiest of memories of my afternoons at Monkland.

As I stood alone looking around at the scene of devastation, it was difficult to comprehend that only a day before the old house had been standing and everything was normal. Tired though I was, I wanted to explore the damage and try to recapture those memories, but Mum and Dad were worried that the bombsite was unsafe and urged me to come no further up the path. I remember naughtily ignoring their pleas. Despite a throbbing and aching leg wound, I was determined to have a last look at some of my old haunts in the garden. Most were strewn with rubble and covered with thick dust, but I could still make out the tree I used to climb and the low wall I used to straddle, pretending to be a cowboy riding on the roof of a train and imitating a scene from a Western film. I had been able to play that game only quite recently, and only after the beautiful wrought iron railings had been removed as part of the War Effort. I had witnessed that 'despicable act of unnecessary vandalism' as Dad called it. Many years later he told me how his pleas to spare the railings had been ignored by the gang dispatched by the authorities to perform the execution. His pleas were met by a sneering rebuff: 'Don't you lot know there's a f****** war on? They iron railings is needed to build Spitfires' (*sic*). Dad's argument that wrought iron was of limited use to an aluminium-bodied aircraft fell on deaf ears. The blow torch was lit and the lance cut its way through the railings, which were dumped unceremoniously onto a large pile. Father later told me that he was aware that this was a clever propaganda exercise to make the public believe that they were helping the war effort in a collective and positive way. In fact, it is doubtful if any of the scrap wrought iron was ever used for the war effort at all.

I think it was the suddenness of events over the past twenty-four hours that had the greatest shock effect on all of us. Since my parents had explained to me that we were at war following the famous broadcast in 1939 by the Prime Minister, Neville Chamberlain, both school and home routines had changed, and to some extent we were prepared for hostilities. There were regular fire drill practice sessions with stirrup pumps and fire buckets. Even at school, we had the regular practice of donning gas masks and going into the dank, smelly air raid shelters which had been built on the former tennis courts in the school playground. The windows of our classroom in the junior school looked over to that playground and while my classmates were busy colouring in and making raffia cards I was intently watching the activity surrounding the barrage balloon and the men dressed in RAF uniform who winched it up and down from the platform of a lorry. Even at my tender age, how I wished I could be part of the grown-ups' war preparations.

The Clydebank blitz had really brought hostilities to my doorstep, and events over the last few hours had seemed unreal. All the excitement with which I as a young lad had greeted the arrival of German bombers had now evaporated. Delayed shock was now setting in, and as I took a last look at Monkland and thought about the damage to our own house in Kelvindale, I simply broke down and sobbed uncontrollably. Seeing my distress, Mum and Dad rushed to comfort me with hugs and an outpouring of pure love. 'Let's go, son, and see how we can start again' Dad said with a reassuring pat on my shoulder. I felt instantly better. Hitler, his henchmen and the might of the Luftwaffe had failed to destroy the spirit of our family. I was determined that never again would anything or anyone stand in my way in what I believed was right and good. I think I had grown up in the past twenty-four hours.

Later I asked my father how he had got through that night, and he said he had remembered a beautiful silver salver which carried the Sharp family crest and our motto, 'dum spiro spero', 'while I breathe I hope'. He knew it was there somewhere under the rubble of his father's house, never to be seen again. 'But I *was* still breathing, and I *did* have hope' he said. 'That was what helped me to carry on.'

My parents were strong, resourceful people and I never doubted that we would survive the war and defeat the evil Nazis. I did not realise then, however, just how the events of those few days in 1941 would direct the course of my life.

CHAPTER TWO

AN ENQUIRING MIND

My father, Russell Sharp, was born in Glasgow in 1900 and attended Glasgow Academy before joining Metropolitan-Vickers, the engineering group, as a trainee in Manchester. His father had been a lawyer, a Justice of the Peace and businessman who had acquired several businesses including sweet factories and a small precision engineering factory. By ancestry the family is German (which is rather ironic, considering the events described in the previous chapter). Originally named Scherp or Scherpe, my antecedents came from the Dresden area, which of course was heavily bombed by the British later in the war; although it is doubtful whether any distant relatives from that branch of the family still exist, I hope that they did not suffer in the way we did in Glasgow.

The Scherps settled in the town of Little Horton in Yorkshire, now part of Bradford, and became quite successful. In the 17th century one of them, John Sharp, was made Dean of Canterbury and later Archbishop of York, the last holder of that title to be entombed there. He must have been a powerful personality, as he was described as a 'vehement preacher whose eyes flamed remarkably'. He held office from 1691 to 1714 and had four children and four grandsons. His son Thomas became Archdeacon of Northumberland and one of Thomas' sons, William Sharp, became a Fellow of the Royal Society and Royal Physician to George III. He spent most of his time studying the King's excretory output, which may have been rather relevant, as porphyria, the disease which is famous for its association with George III, can be diagnosed through dark urine. My distant ancestor might have been on to the problem, although it was not conclusively diagnosed until long after the King's death.

There is a painting of the Sharp family by Johann Zoffany in the National Portrait Gallery in London which I have often visited. It is entitled 'The Family of William Sharp, Musical Party on the Thames'. Painted around 1780, it was commissioned by William Sharp, who stands at the helm of the family barge wearing his court uniform of the House of Windsor. It shows a large number of Sharps all playing on board their barge. Some of the instruments depicted in the painting are of great interest to musical historians. They were a highly musical family and clearly a very outgoing one; they regularly used to give concerts at weekends by travelling up and down the river Thames on William's barge.

One of William's brothers was an engineer, which perhaps points the way to the family inclination which developed later. Some of the Sharps moved to Scotland, although I believe I am descended from another branch which remained in Yorkshire. More recently a member of the Kent branch founded the Sharp's Toffee company, and with this and my grandfather's involvement in the confectionary business I was known at school as 'Toffee' Sharp - I still am, by my few surviving old school chums.

In 1933 my father married my mother, Mabel Watt-Balderston, who also came from an engineering family; her grandfather was Alexander Watt, one of the large family which produced James Watt, the inventor of the steam engine. Alexander Watt, with four other businessmen, raised capital to found a large steel company, which later led to the massive expansion of iron and steel works in Scotland. He also installed my maternal grandfather on the board of a successful iron foundry in Paisley, so the engineering tradition of my mother's side of the family was strong.

I was an only child, and my father never doubted that I would be a boy. He also rather assumed I would become an engineer like himself. He had become a senior manager at Metropolitan-Vickers and the plan was that he would eventually take over the engineering side of one of grandfather Sharp's business acquisitions (a small engineering and specialised welding company on Clydeside). During his trainee days he had studied and become a member of the Institute of Welding, all in preparation for the future. But the war put paid to that, and by the time the German bombers were finished there was nothing much left to take over. He remained on the managerial side of Metrovick until he retired in 1958.

Believing that the Scots were the finest engineers in the world, Dad wanted to make sure I was born Scottish, and for this reason my mother was rushed back across the border from England for the birth. She however had a different version of the event, claiming that the real reason was to make sure I would qualify to play rugby for Scotland! My father was a great rugby enthusiast, having played for Glasgow Academicals and West of Scotland rugby clubs; he had had a trial for a cap and would have given anything to play for Scotland, but hadn't made it. Like many fathers, he hoped his son would go on to achieve some of his own ambitions. In the event, although I shared his love of rugby and other team sports, I never achieved anything like his standards and had to content myself watching the Calcutta Cup and other Internationals at Murrayfield from the stand.

Even before the events of the war I seemed to have developed a great interest in machinery, and apparently I had an insatiable appetite for knowledge of how things work. My first real introduction to this, to me, exciting new world of engineering came in 1938 with the Empire Exhibition held in Bellahouston Park in Glasgow. For months beforehand my father had talked excitedly about that forthcoming event, and with his company Metrovick displaying in the Engineering Pavilion, the promise of seeing real engines and models of ships built on the Clyde really whetted my appetite. I just couldn't wait to be taken to the exhibition.

The big day eventually came, and although I was only three at the time I can still remember the excitement when Mum and I arrived at the entrance gates to the Exhibition Park. There in front of us were massive white buildings, a gleaming tower up on the hill, lots of fountains and waterfalls, flags of all colours flying from masts and hordes of people strolling down avenues between the exhibition buildings. It was simply a wonderland for a young lad like me and I wanted to look at everything, although time was short and

Mum wanted to get me moving on to visit the Engineering Pavilion. On the way I spotted a funfair and was so disappointed that I was too young to be allowed on one of the fairground rides – fighter aeroplanes that 'flew' round in a circle at the end of long arms. Oh how I would have loved to be in the cockpit of one of these! To my young eyes this captured all the thrill of flying. Although I didn't know it at the time, it was perhaps this disappointment that gave me an early determination to fly aeroplanes one day.

Just as Dad had promised, the engineering displays were a feast for very young eyes. There were models of ships built on the Clyde, ships' engines galore and controls and motors for tramcars and railway engines. Noting my interest in the model of the new Coronation Tramcar, which had very recently replaced the ageing Standard tram in Glasgow, one of Dad's colleagues asked me if I would like to see the real thing. He knew one would be parked close to the entrance to the Exhibition Park. Of course I jumped at the chance. I remember how I gasped in admiration as I saw it standing there gleaming in its new livery of orange and green, with the Glasgow Corporation coat of arms emblazoned on its side. It was empty, waiting for passengers to flood out from the Exhibition.

I was shown upstairs, downstairs and all over the passenger compartment, but the highlight of the visit came when we went into the driving cabin. I had to be lifted up by the driver to have a pretend shot at the controls. This, the driver said, entitled me to a tin badge, which he produced from a box in his cabin. Specially made for young visitors to the Transport Pavilion, it proclaimed that I was now officially a 'Junior Tramcar Driver'. That badge was kept among my childhood box of treasures for a long time.

Mum told me later that I had asked endless questions of the poor driver, one of which was why there was a strange contraption in front of the tramcar. He apparently tried his best to explain that it was called a 'cowcatcher', but it was much later that Dad gave an explanation that my very young mind could understand. It arose, he said, from the need for American railroad locomotives crossing the prairies to have something to prevent cattle from getting under the wheels and derailing the train. This cleared up something which had puzzled my young mind since my visit, as I had never seen any cows on the streets of Glasgow!

After that visit, I told my father that all I wanted to be when I grew up was a tram or train driver, but he went to great pains to point out that engineering would be a much more rewarding career. I am sure that when he finally persuaded me to change my ideas he must have felt his plans for my future career were heading in, as he saw it, the right direction.

For the next two or three years I grew up in our house in Kelvindale and attended junior school at Glasgow Academy. It was a short tramcar ride of four stops to Kelvinbridge. I greatly enjoyed these early junior school days and loved learning new things and having new adventures. Even after war was declared in 1939, preparations for hostilities fascinated me, and I enjoyed watching public air raid shelters being built and emergency water tanks being placed along the route to school. What a thrill it was to see Bren gun carriers and the occasional tank coming in convoy up Great Western Road, their caterpillar tracks making a dreadful noise on the road surface; I watched camouflage-painted army lorries carrying equipment needed for the war effort as they passed the bottom of our road en route to their military destinations. Concrete pill boxes were constructed and ready-to-prime road mines placed strategically to thwart any invasion of the City by enemy tanks. Again came the endless questions as my poor parents tried to meet the cravings of my inquisitive mind.

Fitting and testing our gas-masks was fun, although I am told I made such a scene by refusing to wear a 'Mickey Mouse' version of the mask designed specially for children. Eventually, I got my way and was equipped with a mask designed for a small adult. That mask lasted me to the end of hostilities, although as usual, my curiosity to see how it worked necessitated several changes of the charcoal filter.

In the two or three more years and before the Clydebank Blitz changed our lives, my interest began to focus on aeroplanes. My maternal grandparents' house was on the edge of Abbotsinch airfield (now Glasgow Airport), where there were aeroplanes of Bomber Command and later a Spitfire squadron. It had become a torpedo training unit, training both RAF and RN crews, so there was a great variety of aeroplanes to be observed from my grandparents' garden. I became quite proficient at aircraft recognition.

As the war progressed, the significance of the preparations and activities I had witnessed became clearer to me, and the destruction of our house during the Clydebank Blitz of 1941 left me in no doubt that war was a serious business that could have terrible consequences.

We escaped the devastation of the bombing by moving north to Dunblane, where we stayed until 1943. At first we stayed with old school friends of my mothers. Father continued to travel by train from Dunblane railway station to the Metrovick office in Glasgow; petrol was rationed and although, because of his work, he got an allocation of E (Essential) Petrol Coupons, he preferred to use public transport whenever he could.

He was appointed as a senior member of the Ministry of Supply and spent days away on test trials of ships and submarine engines on the Clyde. Mum always knew that when he returned exhausted his work had been demanding, dangerous or both. He never talked about his work and only years later did we extract bit by bit just a few of his wartime activities. After the war, he refused an honour for his efforts, believing that he was doing nothing more than his duty to his King and Country and that there were far more deserving people. That was typical of Dad's unassuming nature, and I have tried to follow his example in my own life and career.

Much to my initial embarrassment, I was sent to the Beacon School for Girls in Bridge of Allan, a few miles south of Dunblane. As a concession to the war effort the school had agreed to take about five or six young boys who like myself had been evacuated to that part of the country or had been taken out of boarding school at the outbreak of the war. I instantly made friends of them and between us we managed to hold our own against the taunts of boys from another school who often met us at the drop-off point for the Alexander's bus which plied between Bridge of Allan and Dunblane. I had been taught by Dad how to defend myself, and this came in handy whenever a scrap broke out between rival lads. Again my pals and I stood our ground and in the end some of the 'enemy' became friends.

Lessons at the Beacon School were not dissimilar to those of the junior school at Glasgow Academy, and this helped to reduce any effects of disruption to learning. We had lots of activities and because of our attendance at a predominantly girls' school the staff arranged for a Wolf Cub pack to be formed. It must have been the smallest cub pack in the world, but I learned so much from our outdoor and indoor activities and from the 'Akela' who was our leader. We gathered potatoes into sacks in the field behind the school; we were helping to 'Dig for Victory' or 'Lend a hand on the land', as the Ministry of Food posters urged us.

Despite the horrors I had seen in the blitz and the deprivations we endured, I was a happy child and was always laughing and having fun. My pals and I would climb trees and I would come home with dirty knees like any other little boy. I had a great appetite for life and was constantly curious, always wanting to know how everything worked. I got into trouble once for poking a knitting needle through the fretwork of the family radio and into the silk behind it to find the little man who was talking, the first signs of a practical interest in broadcasting which would develop later.

I became particularly friendly with a boy called Robert, a lad of my own age with whom I shared many interests. He was also an energetic and enterprising lad. His father owned a large furniture store in Stirling, although they lived near us in Dunblane.

With the help of both fathers we constructed a go-cart (or 'bogey' in Scots vernacular). It was made out of planks of wood, a soapbox and some second-hand pram wheels which Mum managed to purchase from a tinker family camped close by. She paid two shillings for them.

Here again my intrinsic experimental engineering skills became apparent, as I added what I believed was a unique way of steering the kart using two wooden levers instead of feet on the axle rod. This enabled two small people (Rob and myself) to sit tandem, and to allow me to steer from behind I rigged up two wooden levers connected to the front axle by string or old washing line.

During the test run all went well until I, as 'test driver', was careering down a steep country lane close to the house when the experimental steering system failed (the string broke). Robert and I were thrown off, fortunately into a soft grassy bank. Rob was unhurt, but during the tumble I think I bashed my nose on something (possibly the back of his head) and it poured blood for quite a long time. Still to this day it gives me problems from time to time. It was a painful and bloody lesson that taught me about the importance of checking and double-checking systems before launching into the unknown.

Dad was sympathetic to my nose injury, as I recall, but forgetting my very young age and inexperience he couldn't help criticise the poor design and choice of a steering system on which, he pointed out, my life might depend. Any kind of bad engineering he considered to be inexcusable. A lesson was learned for the future.

Mum didn't think much of it either. In her early days she had raced MG motor cars and was proud of having tested racers on the Brooklands circuit, some of them fitted with crankshafts made in her father's foundry. I think she was secretly quite delighted that I might have inherited some of her enterprising spirit. It probably evoked memories of her own childhood when she had borrowed her brother's Indian model motorcycle and terrorised the Paisley residents with her antics.

One good thing emerged from that incident. The elderly farmer who witnessed and helped those two wee boys on their go-kart turned out to be an old acquaintance of my parents. Later he showed Robert and me his old cars lying rather neglected in a barn. One was an old Argyll car (made I think in Scotland) and the other, in a state of disrepair, was a Stanley steam car which he was trying to get running again (in order to beat petrol rationing). I know he did eventually succeed, because I was nearly frightened out my wits one misty morning by the car hissing steam and puffing up the incline down which Robert and I had come to grief, the driver engulfed in a cloud of steam. I don't know whether he ever got the car fully roadworthy or was able to use it on the road, or what became of it, but it was a stalwart effort.

There was even less approval for another experiment I carried out when I tried to jump off the garage roof of the Dunblane house using a large golfing umbrella as a parachute. Its inefficiency at breaking my fall became suddenly apparent. I landed with a jolt onto a cold frame which our family friends used to grow lettuces and other kitchen produce. Fortunately only my pride was hurt on that occasion and with no harm done, I was forgiven. It was quickly pointed out that had I struck or landed on a nearby beehive, things might have been very different!

Our time in Dunblane came to an end when the threat from the bombing declined. My parents bought a house in the Gartconnel district of Bearsden (a leafy suburb of Glasgow at that time), and I rejoined my old classmates in the junior school at Glasgow Academy. For the moment my experimenting and adventuring were put to one side as I tried to catch up with some of the lessons I had missed during the Dunblane days. But it wouldn't be long before they emerged once again, once we had settled into our new abode.

At last the war and the hostilities came to an end. In May 1945 we celebrated VE (Victory in Europe) Day. The celebrations were wonderful, and people in the neighbourhood danced and sang in the streets. A near neighbour of ours managed to get hold of dozens of emergency flares which had been made for use by downed airman needing to be rescued. It was the first time I had seen anything resembling fireworks, and to see the evening sky lit up with coloured flares was pure magic. We lit bonfires on the hill in front of our house and people somehow managed to find enough food and other goodies despite the food restrictions. It was my first experience of eating al fresco. People waved flags, church bells rang out again and spirits soared. Later we watched newsreels at the cinema and saw similar celebrations in London and many other cities throughout Britain. We had won through.

VJ Day (Victory over Japan) was a much more subdued affair, although it signalled the final end to hostilities. We now all longed to get back to normal. We were at last able to enjoy the first holiday we had had as a family since the outbreak. We stayed in a country hotel in Torphins, near Aberdeen, Dad having saved up enough petrol coupons to drive us up there in his car. People across the country were joyous that the war was over, and we all expected food rationing to end and supplies to be restored. It was not to be; rationing continued, as it turned out, right into the 1950s. Only three weeks after

VE day, the food ration was actually cut. Everything was difficult to get and there were always long queues at our local shops in Bearsden for bread and potatoes. Very strange food substitutes appeared on the shelves. Whale and horsemeat were used as additives to eke out the meagre meat rations, while the memory of 'snoek', a peculiar and to most people revolting tinned fish from South Africa, still evokes unpleasant memories.

Sweets were still on ration and our family ration book only allowed a tiny bag of sweets or a small bar of chocolate. It was a disappointment for a family like ours, used to an endless supply from our factories. I think we all had an obsession about food and longed for things like bananas and real ice cream. As sweet-hungry youngsters we were still able to obtain cinnamon sticks from pre-war stocks in chemist shops. Sometimes we would chew them, or for variety we would light one end and smoke them. Occasionally we could buy so-called 'cigarette sweets', white chews in the shape of a real cigarette with one end coloured red to make them look real. Goodness knows how many young lads were drawn into cigarette smoking through these early sweet substitutes. For some, liquorice sticks dipped into a bag of sherbet helped to satisfy the craving for sweet things, although the laxative effect of that confection was a price that had to be paid. Food substitutes seemed to be the order of the day. As always I tried to adapt a recipe I had read in a newspaper and tried to make ersatz bananas by soaking boiled parsnips in a so-called banana essence. It tasted awful, but then nobody of our age knew what a banana looked like, far less tasted like. That was until a boy in my class brought in a banana which a relative had brought back with him on leave from the Army. It was short and stumpy and an ugly green colour, not a bit like the pictures of the beautiful, gently-curved bright yellow fruit we used to see advertising Fyffes' bananas on old railway station hoardings. We all longed to have a taste of it, but our form mistress decided the fairest thing would be to put it up for auction – the proceeds would go to a school-supported charity for the returning war-wounded.

I joined in the bidding, which rapidly rose to ridiculous heights. My final bid of ten shillings (a great deal of money in those days) was just beaten by the boy sitting at the next desk to me. He was an unpopular and cocky little lad who refused to share his trophy and made us watch him as he peeled the skin back and slowly and deliberately savoured the taste of the fruit.

At this point a boy at the back of the class found this too much to bear. He rushed down between the desks, knocking the banana out of its owner's hand and spreading it over the floor. There was an almighty scramble to try and retrieve what parts of the now mushy fruit had not been trampled on. The winner of the auction, having pledged his bid money, managed to retrieve only a small part of the prize he had won.

The rest of us had to wait until the 'banana boats' returned to our shores before we knew what we had missed for all those war years. When I told my parents about my failed attempt to buy the banana, they almost had pink fits, but were relieved that they wouldn't have to honour the bid. I got a flaming row from Dad and a lecture on the value of money. It was another lesson I learned.

My father was very good at telling stories, and one of his subjects was flying. He used to tell me in great detail about Alcock and Brown's pioneering transatlantic flight in a modified Vickers Vimy bomber in 1919, with the bomb carriers replaced by enough tanks to carry 865 gallons of fuel. Father actually knew Arthur Whitten Brown, a Glaswegian like him, and had worked with him. I used to think that was marvellous, to think of those brave men flying all that way for sixteen hours across three thousand miles of ocean to win honour and fame. I would re-enact it at home, with a table and chairs as the plane, the carpet as the blue sea and the curtains to represent fog.

Even at that age the one thing that interested me even more than the engineering dimension was the aviators, and how they had endured it all. Father told of the great tension when communication with Alcock and Brown was cut off and it was feared that they had been lost at sea; in fact their radio had packed up. I wondered how those brave men had stayed awake and coped with the stress and the discomfort. It was the beginning of an interest that would develop a great deal further.

Thanks to Alcock and Brown and Dad's involvement with the Vickers Vimy, I developed an early fascination for aircraft and flying. It helped that my mother's family home in Paisley was near Abbotsinch Airfield. My favourite reading in those days, unsurprisingly, was the Biggles books of Captain W E Johns.

Soon after the war I progressed to the senior school. Teaching was not good at the time. Old, tired schoolmasters had held the school together when the younger ones were away at war. I did however make many friends with whom I have remained friendly all my life. We would make fun of some of the masters, as boys do – I remember 'Shorty' Gilmour, 'Dick'

Tate and 'Baggy' Aston. Later a younger gym master joined the staff, Henry U'ren, who did not need a nickname.

One teacher we did not make fun of in senior school was Katy 'Lentils' Gentles. She was a formidable mistress who taught younger classes in senior school. She wore a black academic gown and had a tawse (Scottish leather strap) hanging beneath her gown, and used it liberally on our hands or bottoms for almost any misdemeanour. However I owe 'Lentils' a great deal for the teaching methods she used, which became the basis for my scientific and research career. She took us out on visits to factories, carpet works, haulage contractors and many others in the days before out-of-classroom activities became commonplace. She insisted on our return that we must investigate all aspects of the work carried out in these workplaces to see what was involved in every task, using the books and encyclopaedias in the school library bookshelves. Then we had to write up a short essay or report on what we had observed. I became quite skilled at taking information and writing a précis, and because of this I won a class prize for my visit reports.

Again the slant I took was the human aspects of the workplace. My ability to précis information stood me in good stead for my later lecturing and broadcasting work. It was also the groundwork for what was to come later and my early introduction to the almost unknown field of occupational medicine –my final goal.

The month of January 1947, when I was eleven, brought the worst winter weather Britain had experienced for decades. Throughout the country, heavy snowfalls blocked roads and railway lines, making travel a near impossibility. Taps froze and water pipes burst. Coal supplies, already low following the war, could not reach the power stations, which were forced to shut down, bringing power cuts and restrictions to thousands of homes.

In Scotland the snowdrifts and freezing temperatures were particularly bad and the route to school quickly became blocked. The school buses were unable to get through and we all rejoiced at this unscheduled holiday. There was fun to be had with snowball fights, sliding on ice runs and skating on hard frozen ponds and lochs. It was a new experience to most of us.

Two of my pals had steerable sledges, one called a 'Flexi Flyer' and the other a 'Yankee Clipper'. They were state-of-the-art toboggans and my friends always won downhill races on the packed snow run we made on a steep hill near our house. I just couldn't compete with them. The crude, unsteerable wooden sledge my much older cousin gave me became the target of sneers.

Enterprising as ever, I decided that I would modify this sledge and beat the lot of them on downhill races. I managed to unearth several pairs of old ice skates which had been my mother's and screwed them on to the wooden runners of the sledge. I even managed to fix another pair to a wooden axle bar, which gave me some steering capability. After several sessions honing the skate runners to perfection and with an additional treatment with candlewax, the sledge was ready for speed trials. It may have looked awful by comparison with the professional ones, but my goodness it simply flew. I won all the races after that and there were no further sneers.

As March of that year approached we experienced very high, almost gale force winds. Again my inventive mind turned to the prospect of harnessing this power to good use. I tried making all kinds of kites from box kite designs which I found in magazines. They didn't work very well. I turned to other simpler designs and they flew better but were quite uncontrollable.

I decided to design my own version, but reversed the anchor point from the inside of the kite to the outside. The creation of four air pockets, rather than one, gave the kite much better lift and I knew then that I was on to a winner. The final model I built from broom handles and some old blackout curtain material we had left after the war. On the first trial run of the new giant kite, the ball of string I used snapped, but I managed to replace this with several clothes lines tied together. It was incredible! The kite soared in the wind to a good height. I nearly lost it, but I hung on for grim death and almost immediately was lifted off my feet. I was actually airborne for the first time in my life, but there was no time to enjoy the flight. I don't know how high I actually reached, not too high I suspect, but I decided it was time to bail out. Fortunately the wind dropped suddenly and the kite sank towards the ground. Just when I thought the time was right, I let go and made a kind of landing on a muddy wet patch. I was unhurt, but that experiment as an eleven-year-old going on twelve started me thinking about how parachutists land without injury and how fliers deal with emergencies in stricken aircraft. It was the beginning of an interest which would dominate my career.

CHAPTER THREE

MR McCABE AND THE TREE OF LIFE

As the years went on and I passed through my teens, thoughts of mechanics and engineering gave way to other priorities. I soon began dating girls. Like most of my generation, I had many short-term girlfriends, on a largely innocent basis. This was the age of birthday parties and school dances. They were a pleasant diversion after the dark, dismal and cheerless wartime days. I loved ballroom and Scottish country dancing and my father paid for lessons at the Alice McEwan School of Dancing in Sauchiehall Street in Glasgow city centre.

Much of the time my chums and I spent drinking Coca Cola and smoking cigarettes up in the balcony of the studio, instead of learning our steps. Alice McEwan herself put a stop to all this with the threat that we wouldn't be taught the Tango, the favourite dance at the time. With more involvement and concentration I got to know all the steps and became quite proficient on the dance floor.

The era of going to dances and charity balls, first with my parents and later in my own right, had started, and I met lots of friends and girlfriends my own age through that. Many a romance started through these.

Most of the early dating however was done on the Alexanders' double-decker bus that plied between Bearsden and Glasgow. Here on the way to and from school we met with the Laurel Bank girls on the top deck, who joined us several stops up the road. One of my greatest school chums, Campbell (Plummy) Duff, fell for a Laurel Bank girl, Janet, he met on the bus. She was to become his future wife and a cordon bleu cook. Perhaps she discovered that the 'stomach was the way to a man's heart'. Campbell and Janet have remained great family friends of ours.

At the time, it was a great puzzle to me how old 'Plummy' and others seemed to attract girls who flocked round them, whereas I seemed to be less successful and had to work hard at dating. The clue to the attraction became evident when the time came for us to join the school Combined Cadet Force (CCF).

Here's how. With my interest in flying I was desperate to join the Air Cadet section. They got to fly in gliders and sometimes an RAF Anson trainer. That attracted me greatly, but places were very limited and although I got on the shortlist when the day of selection came I had to miss out, as I was in detention. I had to make do with the Army Section, although for a bit of variety I joined the Corps pipe band and learned to play the tenor drum (I tried the bagpipes but just couldn't hack them).

On the bus into school it became obvious that what the girls liked was the uniform. Campbell Duff scored because he was in naval uniform and the girls threw themselves at him. I thought I too had scored when I went on the bus in my full pipe-band regalia of kilt, tunic, plaid, sporran, white spats, Glengarry bonnet and various highland adornments. I felt like the bee's knees and thought I must have looked a million dollars. Sure enough, the Laurel Bank girls flocked round me like bees to a honey pot. Great, I thought, until I soon discovered when the kilt lifting began that the attraction was not me, but the old burning question of what underwear I might or might not be wearing under the kilt!

After that I accepted a lift to school in Dad's car whenever there was a pipe band parade. Thereby modesty was preserved and the age-old question remained firmly under wraps!

Still, I wasn't to be beaten, and for a very short time I joined the others in the Naval Section. I felt Fleet Air Arm and naval aviation might just fill the gap and meet my longing to fly. It didn't, and I did not enjoy learning how to tie knots (bowline on a bight, reef knots etc) under the stern eye of Chief Petty Officer Hoskins. Nor did I enjoy 'sea days' aboard HMS *Blackburn*, an RNVR vessel we used for exercises in the Firth of Clyde. Seagoing was no match for flying, I thought, although I had not in fact yet had the opportunity to fly an aircraft. I did enjoy signalling with semaphore flags in the playground, but one of my naval section chums broke the rules by signalling awful obscene messages to another boy without realising that an ex-Wren officer living opposite the playground could also read them. A complaint was made to the Rector and all members of naval section were punished by extra duties. Paper Aldis lamps and Morse code as a replacement actually suited me, as it was closer to air navigation and signalling.

Fed up with it all, I rejoined the Army section, where I was promoted to corporal and began to enjoy my School Corps once again. Strangely I enjoyed the CCF Field Days at Mugdock Moor close to Milngavie and north of Glasgow. There in muddy fields and often in pouring rain we practised a variety of army manoeuvres and exercises. Despite the discomfort and exhaustion I enjoyed these days out of the classroom, which were a welcome application of the things we had been taught by our instructors. I became proficient in rifle shooting and gained the coveted 'rifle badge' on my uniform sleeve, sitting next to the badge awarded for completion of Certificate A parts one and two. This helped towards my promotion and I owed much to my Dad, who used to take me out on some of the shooting parties he attended.

In these earlier years, schoolwork seemed to drag on and on in what I felt was an endless monotony, relieved from time to time by games and activities with the Science Club and Photographic Club. There were visits to the Western Baths, where I learned to swim using the breast stroke, but I never seemed to master what was then referred to as the 'American crawl'. My early interests in radio broadcasting also took me into drama, and I joined the Globe Players, where we put on several Shakespeare plays and in a lighter vein the annual Christmas concerts. The latter gave me a reasonably legitimate excuse to mimic our teachers. It was popular amongst my classmates but a little less popular with some of the older and more staid masters, who seemingly couldn't take a joke.

As the time approached for me to leave school, I began to focus my thoughts on my career. In those days, in the early 1950s, career advice was not generally available, and to be offered a career interview was a rarity. As often as not your choice of job still depended on your background and circumstances. If you had been born into a coal-mining family, it was down the mine for you; if you were a farmer's son you would more than likely take up agriculture. Although thoughts of medicine as a career had been sparked off by my experience of the Blitz, I was still a little uncertain exactly what career pathway I would take - until, that is, I met Mr McCabe.

I was about sixteen years old at the time and still in the fifth form. Mr McCabe (I never knew his first name or where he was from) was a dour and mildly eccentric retired schoolmaster, a tall thin man with a long nose and small round steel-rimmed spectacles and a kind of shabby academic look about him. He was the sort of person you would expect to see sitting at a desk, quill pen in hand, in a dimly-lit Dickensian office. He was one of a small group invited every year by the Rector to dispense wisdom and advice about our future careers. I was one of those who had volunteered to see him,

Mr McCabe must have been blessed with a very unusual gift, I thought, because after ten minutes during which we talked about my hobbies, interests and general aspects of my life, he was able to come up with a firm suggestion for a career which he considered suited to my abilities and personality.

'Have you thought about peach-canning?' he said. He looked at me with piercing eyes, waiting for a reaction.

'*Peach*-canning?' I repeated his words, hoping that he would not detect the incredulity in my voice.

'Well, not *just* peaches' he continued. 'Your work might

include apricots, and possibly pears as well. There are some excellent opportunities for a worthwhile career in fruit processing in South Africa.'

I could not believe what I was hearing. There were no signs that he was being anything other than serious as he went on to paint a picture of the idyllic life I could look forward to if I entered upon a career in the canning of fruit. I could be processing peaches in the morning, and in the afternoon I could be swimming in a warm blue sea or relaxing on a warm, sunny South African beach. He made it sound like a way of life which no one in their right mind could possibly resist.

'Well, I hadn't actually thought about that as a career' I replied, beginning to feel the whole conversation was becoming just a little ridiculous. Was he playing games with me, I wondered?

'I am hoping to study medicine, and next year I'll be applying for a place in Medical School at Glasgow University' I told him.

'Ah, you want to be a doctor.' Mr McCabe paused thoughtfully for a few seconds. Then he leaned forward, his eyes glinting behind his spectacles. Without a trace of a smile, he said 'Then it has to be patients, not peaches, for you, young man?'

I nodded, forcing a weak smile. He continued in a typically schoolmaster voice. 'What brought you to that choice of career, my boy? Do you have a parent or relative who's a doctor?'

I replied in the negative. Having ascertained that there were no doctors in my family, he seemed to want to probe a little further. 'When and what decided you to join the noble profession?' he enquired loftily.

I was a bit thrown by the question, as I had not really thought much about it, but I answered as truthfully as I could. 'I've wanted to be a doctor for as long as I can remember' I said. 'And yes, there was an experience which might have helped me to confirm that decision, in the war. I've also read as many medical books as I can. I enjoyed *The Microbe Hunters* and a book about the life of Marie Curie, and I really want to be like these doctors and make scientific discoveries. I am quite attracted to the research and scientific side of medicine.'

I paused for a moment. 'And then there's broadcasting' I added. 'My father has been involved in that, and it interests me too.'

'Good!' he said. 'We are beginning to get somewhere. You have already identified the aspects of medicine which you feel might be meaningful and rewarding, and that is important. You are more likely to succeed in a career you feel passionate about.'

He looked straight at me. 'Any particular aspects of medicine you might have thought about - say a specialized branch of medicine or surgery?'

I hesitated for a moment and then blurted out 'Flying, sir - I love everything about aeroplanes. If possible I would love to combine flying with medicine.'

My reply seemed to take him aback, and he leaned back in his chair, looking thoughtful. He would surely think I had been reading too many Biggles books. I didn't dare mention that as a younger boy I had also enjoyed *Doctor Dolittle In The Moon*, as I'm sure he would have thought that was going a little too far into my flights of fancy.

'I know it sounds a bit strange,' I continued almost

apologetically, 'but these are my real interests and passions. Medicine, flying and broadcasting.'

His face didn't move a muscle. 'So,' he said. 'For you it is neither peaches nor patients you want to look after, but pilots. You want, in fact, to be a research flying doctor. An interesting choice.'

He sat forward in his chair and pointedly closed the file containing all my old school results and reports. 'That's the end of that' I thought. 'He must think I'm totally crazy.'

After a brief pause in the conversation, he continued, 'You are choosing a career, my boy, with a long and difficult road ahead and you must be very sure - very sure indeed - that you are making the right decision. Remember, the choice you make is going to affect your life and the lives of any family you might have in the future. It might help you to choose wisely if you could make a note of projects or topics that excite your imagination. Reflect on stories of people you admire and ask yourself why certain activities make you happy and contented. Keep asking yourself what you want from your life and career. In that way your choice will be the right one for you.'

With that he stood up from his desk, indicating that we had come to the end of my allotted time. I thanked him for his advice and started to make for the classroom door. But before I could reach it, Mr McCabe spoke again. Almost as an afterthought, he added, 'It might not be a bad idea for you to jot down on paper all the experiences, influences and anything else which may have helped you to reach your career decision. Write down whatever you have in mind, no matter how improbable it seems. And if you can, assign an importance to each item on the list - it will help to point you in the right direction. Also, if you're ever asked about your choice, these notes will help to jog your memory.'

Clearly he was thinking about the selection interview for a place in medical school which I would face in a year or so. They always asked the same questions: 'Why do you want to be a doctor?' and 'What branch of medicine attracts you the most?' They would expect an answer beyond the usual stock one trotted out by most candidates.

I returned to my classroom, where I shared my experiences of the careers advice session with my classmates. It seemed that all had been initially questioned on their views of a bizarre choice of occupation or career. Most thought Mr McCabe somewhat eccentric and considered his advice to be less than useful to them. I took a slightly different view. When I thought about the advice I had received and the words of wisdom he had given me, I realized that this was exactly what Mr McCabe had wanted me to do; to stop and think about my career choice. That strange suggestion of peach canning was of course a clever device to make me do so. He was a remarkable man.

Mr McCabe also told me to go away and draw my own personal tree of life. Then I should complete it with branches representing each of the things I wanted to do. I drew up my tree as suggested, and of course the central branch was medicine, with others for flying, science and broadcasting.

That career interview helped me to collect together my thoughts for a career. My experiences in the blitz had sparked off the idea of a medical career. Miss 'Lentils' Gentles had introduced me to techniques of studying and the possible application of science to the workforce and the workplace. Through the tales of Alcock and Brown and their epic transatlantic crossing, my father had helped me to turn my thoughts to helping aviators to cope with the demands and hazards of flying. My career pathway was now beginning to take shape, and I started to look forward to the time when I could get started.

By the time I had finished the fifth form I had managed to do reasonably well in the Higher Leaving Certificate exams and had obtained the necessary qualifications to gain a place at university. I felt that now I was well on my way to my chosen career and eagerly completed an application to study Medicine at Glasgow University.

I was made a School Prefect, which gave me a much larger measure of freedom and authority. It was a tradition that new prefects were given an initiation task. In my case the Head Prefect gave me the task of trying to identify the culprit who had scribbled the letter 'F' in front of the word 'ART' engraved on the frosted window above the door of the Art Room. Everyone knew it was there and had probably been so for many years. All attempts by the School Janitor to erase it had apparently been fruitless. Whenever it was cleaned off the window a new letter 'F' was scrawled back on the pane, and a new culprit had to be identified and punished if caught. Although I had my suspicions, I never actually found the culprit and was quite glad I hadn't succeeded in my task, as it was the kind of thing I might have done myself in my slightly younger and wilder days.

For the remaining time as a prefect I was tasked with patrolling the labyrinth of the old air-raid shelters trying to catch boys smoking during the break. I was rather more successful in this task, as I knew from my own experiences just where the best places were to have a smoke undetected. It was a case of 'set a thief to catch a thief,' but I usually turned a blind eye and let the smokers escape.

I really enjoyed those final years at school. Although they were perhaps my happiest time at school, there was one final 'fly in the ointment' and a serious obstacle that threatened to ruin my planned career in medicine - the requirement for boys of my age to carry out a period of National Service. At first I wasn't too despondent, knowing that if my application to study medicine was successful I would be exempt from service. Just in case it wasn't successful I accepted the fact that if it had to be, I could always try for the RAF and even get the chance of flying. There was always another possibility - that of joining the Fleet Air Arm and flying from Royal Navy aircraft carriers. That hope was shattered when reports from other hopeful applicants to these services were being rejected in favour of infantry soldiering. The Korean War was building up and army ground forces were the priority. It didn't help my despondency to hear soon afterwards that Jimmy Crowe, the lad two years ahead of me who taught me drumming, had been killed in action out in Korea. I was particularly cut up about Jimmy's death.

The compulsory registration and medical examination for National Service recruits was held in a nearby drill hall belonging to the Highland Light Infantry based at Maryhill Barracks. I got my call-up papers and was instructed to attend on a certain day and time. The first part of the interview by three officers was farcical. They were not interested in anything I had done or any of my abilities and ambitions. All it seemed they wanted was 'cannon fodder' with no regard for anyone's preferences.

The medical examination too was strange. I was examined and prodded from top to toe by the Medical Officer, my eyesight and hearing were tested and finally I was asked to provide a sample of urine for testing. Try as I might I just wasn't able to oblige. It was not assisted by the fact that I was standing outside the cubicle wearing only my underwear and in an open hall crowded with fellow applicants. I could see that the officer in the next cubicle was becoming impatient and the caretaker, who was clearly out of his depth, was hurrying me on and urging me to provide my specimen.

Finally, after a long delay during which I thought about fountains and running water, I managed to produce a pathetic but just adequate quantity of urine. The caretaker held the specimen up to the light, and without even a glance at the test reagents laid out on his table said, 'You've had no trouble with your kidneys, have you son?'

'Not as far as I am aware' I replied, and my hard-won specimen was thrown into a bucket. I was propelled into the next cubicle for completion of paperwork. That was it. I was pronounced fit and told to wait for the official papers to arrive in the post. They weren't interested in hearing that I hoped to get deferment if my application for Medical School was accepted. I could only hope and pray.

I was in Switzerland with a school party when my parents sent me a telegram telling me I had obtained my place at university. It was a great relief that I would be deferred from National Service, but I was rather sorry for those of my classmates who were not so lucky.

I went up in October 1952. It was then a six-year course and I continued to live at home, as there was no need to seek student lodgings. I regret that slightly now, as I have realised that moving away from home and being plunged into the outside world is an essential part of further education.

It didn't stop me, however, from having a good time. In my first year I joined just about every society and student club activity I could. I really enjoyed the student life of dances and parties during that first year. I still slightly envied the few former school classmates who had gone up to Oxford and Cambridge and come home in the vacation with tales of jolly japes and riotous rag weeks in their student life.

My attempt to emulate the Oxbridge student life took its toll. For the first time I failed an exam – the end of the year professional exam in organic chemistry - although fortunately, a successful re-sit over the summer vacation allowed me to progress into my second year. It was a near thing, and it taught me not to try to burn the candle at both ends.

After that I took lectures and classes much more seriously and rationed the time I spent on social activities, which included the rounds of friends' twenty-first birthday parties. I focused on the aim of obtaining my medical degree as soon as possible and using it as the starting point for a future career pathway.

My first motorised transport had been a BSA Bantam 125cc motorcycle, which I ran when I was in the sixth form at school. The wheels had a habit of getting stuck in the tram lines, and on one occasion a wheel became so firmly lodged in the track that I thought I would finish up in the depot! I had great fun on that little motorcycle and used to race the Post Office telegraph lads, who had the same model but with postbox-red paintwork. A swerve to avoid a crash into the back of another vehicle soon put a stop to these capers. I was catapulted off the bike and onto the road with an almighty thump and slid to a stop in a roadside gutter. My thick leather riding coat took most of the abrasion of the skid, but although I was unhurt the motorbike was badly damaged and almost beyond repair. I sold it more or less for scrap.

I persuaded Dad that four wheels would be safer than two, and when I started at university my father helped me to buy my first car - an ex-army Austin Eight. It had belonged to an army major who had used it as his staff car in the Libyan desert in WW2. After the war it had been 'civilianised', painted grey and the hood replaced with a very smart maroon soft top, removable door side panels with a flap opening and celluloid side and rear windows. It was extremely plain, with no brightwork chromium whatsoever. My father chose this deliberately basic model so that I could get to know the mechanics and working parts. I stripped that poor car down almost to its components, and it taught me car maintenance to a much higher level than I would otherwise have achieved.

Having four wheels was a luxury after the Bantam. No more freezings and soakings on wet days or skidding on slippery cobbled streets, and no more struggling to keep the bike's narrow wheels out of the tram rails.

Having a car, however odd and utilitarian, as a student was a luxury, but it did make me popular with friends needing lifts to parties and dances. It was also useful later on, as it allowed me to avoid public transport and got me on time to outlying hospitals for classes and tutorials. No surprise, I'm sure, that I just couldn't resist modifying the engine, polishing the ports and tweaking just about everything I could to make the car go faster. It must have been the fastest Austin Eight in the country, but the penalty was a massive increase in petrol consumption which my allowance couldn't meet (even with petrol at three shillings and sixpence a gallon). It had to be de-tuned rather smartly.

It was then that I quite literally ran into an old school friend, Arthur Ferns. He was studying Engineering at Glasgow University and our reunion happened as I was driving down University Avenue, late for a class, with Arthur ahead of me. The brakes of my Austin were to say the least a little 'spongy', and when the car in front of him forced Arthur to come to a sudden stop, I ran into the back of his pride and joy - a lovely 1938 classic two-seater MG TB. The MG fared worse than my 'tank' and Arthur was out of the car like a shot to inspect the damage. His face was like thunder, but it changed suddenly when he realised who it was that had caused the damage. We both turned on the poor female lecturer in the car in front, who apologised for her sudden braking, though as a true 'gentleman' I admitted to being the real cause of the shunt and we all departed amicably.

Arthur and his family have remained very dear friends of our family to this day and although we still regularly keep in touch with each other the subject of the incident is never discussed!

After a long six years of study I eventually qualified in 1958. I think this put paid to any lingering doubts my parents might have had about my choice of career. My father had greatly admired the achievements of a works doctor who had introduced industrial health practice, then unknown, in the early Metrovick days. The fact that the doctor was also a qualified engineer helped. My father was happy to recognise that I had made the right choice in entering the medical profession, and he was very proud.

As for me, my only regret was my inability to join the

University Air Squadron. They were giving first priority to potential recruits to the RAF for flying training and were unwilling to fill precious places with medical students who they felt would probably never fly aeroplanes in their lives.

Instead I kept up my interest in aviation by reading every flying magazine I could get hold of. I took a special interest in the new aircraft coming off the production line and entering service with the airlines. Military aircraft at the Farnborough Air Show were of special interest to me and I was thrilled to watch highlights of the event and the many thrilling air displays on Pathé and Gaumont British newsreels at our local cinema.

When it was released in 1956, the film *Reach for the Sky* was a tremendous inspiration and I watched it two or three times when it came to our local cinema. It told the remarkable true story of Douglas Bader, an RAF pilot who overcame every obstacle to pursue the flying career he wanted. Bader was a young and ambitious pilot who lost both his legs in a plane crash. As his service colleagues prepared for his devastation they were to find a determination in him that refused to be changed by the accident. His re-entry to the RAF led to the remarkable flying exploits in World War Two which made him famous. I so admired the courage and determination that enabled Douglas Bader to face and overcome near impossible odds. He immediately became my hero. Little did I know that I would one day meet him.

I was also particularly moved by the Comet disasters which had occurred two years previously as a result of explosive loss of cabin pressure. I read and admired the experimental and detective work of the Royal Aircraft Establishment (RAE), which enabled investigators to identify the underlying cause - metal fatigue - which had led to the accident. This gave me my first interest in flight safety and ways of protecting aircrew and passengers from loss of cabin pressure when flying at high altitude. By now physiology, and particularly aviation physiology, was very much my favourite subject and my aim for the future.

The next step was to do the two six-month house jobs which are still standard in medical training, one a surgical job at the Glasgow Western Infirmary and the other in the children's department at Raigmore Hospital in Inverness.

When I started out on my first House Officer post it felt good to be a 'proper' doctor at last and be treated as such by the nurses and staff of the surgical ward. It was a residency position and I was provided with accommodation in the hospital itself. To a young and recent student this was luxury. My rooms consisted of a bedroom, bathroom en suite and a pleasant lounge with a coal fire that was kept alight constantly.

The work was exceptionally hard, with ward rounds every morning accompanying the surgeons, ward sister and her nursing staff. Then it was into the operating theatre to assist the Consultant, Eric Gerstenberg, with his list for the day. Sometimes these operating sessions would stretch well into the afternoon and I was always worried that this would interfere with my afternoon rounds when I was expected to write up case notes, take endless blood samples for testing and generally put into action the instructions given by my consultants. As often as not it meant a trip down to the blood bank to cross-match blood for transfusion or speedily set up a drip on an ill patient. This was quite a major problem where the patient was in shock and veins were collapsed and difficult to access. By sheer force of numbers, carrying out these procedures stood me in very good stead for research work I carried out in the future.

On nights when our ward was on call for emergency and casualty admissions, there was barely enough time to join my fellow house doctors and grab an evening meal in the staff dining room. If I was lucky I would join the others in the doctors' lounge, where we would listen to *The Goon Show* on an old wireless set which had seen better days. It was a new style of comedy and we all became hooked on this and *Top of the Pops*. Such diversions from the intense and serious work of the hospital were essential, although an uninterrupted evening or an unbroken night's sleep was a rarity.

One of the commonest nocturnal interruptions was a blocked intravenous needle in the blood or saline transfusion sets. In those days infusion sets consisted of a glass bottle suspended from a metal stand and a length of rubber tubing running to the needle, which was inserted into a vein in the patient's arm. I was constantly being wakened at night to change a needle or unblock the system when in the darkness of the night ward the nurses hadn't noticed that the infusion bottle had run out. It usually took ages to put right. This was a regular source of sleep deprivation and resulting sleep debt, and it often had a knock-on effect for the following day's work.

As usual, I decided to tackle this problem myself and designed and built an alarm system which detected when the bottle was nearly empty. The system worked well and triggered a flashing red light on top of the drip stand which the nurses could see from their night station. They were then able to change the bottle before it ran out, and this brought a welcome reduction to my nights of interrupted sleep.

My gadgetry and tinkering had an even more interesting and extraordinary outcome which in many ways had an influence on my future career - I met the renowned and highly respected Professor of Obstetrics and Gynaecology, Ian Donald.

It was when I was building my transfusion alarm gadget that Professor Donald happened to notice the light on in my lounge one evening. Through the door into the corridor he spotted me tinkering with screwdrivers, circuit boards, wiring and spring balances. He was instantly curious to know what I was doing. I think he was intrigued that a young house doctor was interested in mechanics and gadgetry. We discussed our mutual ideas of how engineering and science might be applied to medicine and I learned a lot from him.

What a thrill it was when he invited me to look at his laboratory, which unknown to me was set up in a hospital room only a few yards further down the corridor. It contained the most extraordinary collection of Dexion racking, wires, cables and switches, one which put my meagre efforts to shame. It was an early experimental model of the ultrasound diagnostic system he had invented for use in his specialty, obstetrics.

From that first and several other exchanges there emerged an extraordinary tale of a man who, in many ways like myself, had an early interest in machinery and making gadgets. His obsession with these apparently earned him the name 'Mad Donald'. But mad he most certainly was not; his early experiments led to the development of ultrasound scanning, a technique which is reliable and safe (unlike the former X-ray procedures) and is now a standard test procedure used during pregnancy (as every mother knows and has pictures to prove it.)

Ian Donald joined the RAF and had a most distinguished career, in which he was decorated for gallantry for rescuing the crew of a burning bomber. His service in the RAF sparked his interest in devices like radar and sonar—techniques developed to detect enemy aircraft and submarines respectively. He was quick to recognise that sonar might be used in medical diagnostics.

His early experiments were carried out in a local engineering firm which used industrial metal flaw detectors. These investigations led Ian to explore the value of ultrasound in diagnosing abdominal tumours. It allowed the doctors to differentiate between those that were serious and those that were simple and less so. Further experiments led to the development of the equipment now in modern use for diagnostic scanning during pregnancy. It was a major breakthrough in medicine, and Ian's experimental work greatly inspired me. He was a man after my own heart and his example convinced me that one day I too should explore the value of combining science and engineering with medicine, as he had done so successfully.

Even at the very start of my own medical career, I tried to use every such opportunity to get ideas for research in the future. It was quite amazing how many people I met and how often the most unlikely situations arose that helped me to do just that.

It wasn't long before yet another opportunity like that came my way. About half way through my surgical house job, I managed to snatch a few days of my leave entitlement and flew out of Prestwick airport on a holiday charter to Copenhagen. It was an opportunity to do some early Christmas shopping and see a bit of Denmark. I found myself staying in the same rather smart hotel as the famous American singer and film star Doris Day. What a thrill it was! I was a great fan of hers and always tried to see her new films as soon as they came to our local cinema. It was therefore a very special moment when I came face to face with the great lady in the hotel lobby one morning. We exchanged only a very short greeting and an even briefer comment on the vagaries of Danish weather, but I will never forget the smile she gave me as she turned and walked away surrounded by the usual bevy of hangers-on. I went quite weak at the knees and felt just a little guilty that I, now a professional man, was behaving like a young schoolboy.

I had some extremely interesting discussions with the American film crew who were over in Denmark with Doris, shooting an episode for a weekly television series where she sang and entertained in various popular holiday destinations. The weather was particularly cold in Copenhagen that winter and although most of the locals, including myself, were muffled up in warm clothing, the film crew had arrived totally unprepared for the cold and wet Danish weather. When I spoke to them in the hotel bar and they learned that I was a doctor, I had to field all kinds of questions on the health effects of cold on people exposed to freezing weather conditions. They had resigned themselves to the fact that cold was one of the occupational hazards that was part of their outside work. At that time I knew little or nothing about the topic, but seized the opportunity to find out more. I eagerly accepted an invitation to observe the 'shoot' and watch the episode being filmed from a bridge over one of the many city canals.

It was cold for us standing on the bridge and must have been even colder for poor Doris. She sang a song written for the episode extolling the joys of summer holidays in Denmark. She performed her song on an open-decked barge as it was towed down the canal. The song went something like this: *'Won't you come with me to wonderful Copenhagen, wonderful Copenhagen by the sea...'* Considering the adverse weather conditions her performance seemed immaculate to my untrained eye, but it had to be repeated several times until the directors and technicians felt they had got it just right. A battery of intensely powerful arc lights gave the impression of a beautiful warm Danish summer, although the actual conditions that morning were far from that. The entire film crew were freezing cold, and poor Doris, who had to endure several takes and retakes clad only in a flimsy summer dress, must have been close to collapsing with hypothermia.

This immediately started me thinking about the effects of cold on the human body and the ways hypothermia might be prevented in downed pilots in cold seas, or in outdoor workers in foul weather conditions. This might just be a fruitful line of research for the future, I thought to myself. But for the moment all such thoughts had to be put to one side. There was work to do in the surgical ward in the Western Infirmary back in Glasgow, and my holiday was nearly over.

I went up for my next six-month house job at Raigmore at the start of 1959 for the medical aspect in the paediatric ward. Three months were spent at Raigmore Hospital itself and a further three months at the Inverness Royal Northern Infirmary on the bank of the river Ness. The work was much less frenetic than my post at the Western Infirmary and I was able to visit my parents in Fortrose, near Inverness, at weekends and take days off. We all had to take our turn at being on call for a full day, attending to any casualties or emergencies that might be brought in to the hospital. I became quite adept at removing fishing flies from anglers fishing on the stretch of the river Ness just in front of the Hospital.

During the winter months several hill-walkers were admitted in various stages of hypothermia. One young lad was brought in who had been separated from his party during a severe snow storm in the Cairngorm Mountain range. He had had to spend a night in freezing conditions and somehow managed to survive until the mountain rescue team arrived. Like many others caught out in similar conditions he had been ill-prepared for his ordeal, having set out in thin clothing and with gym shoes instead of proper climbing boots on his feet. With intensive care nursing he suffered no serious after-effects. He was lucky to have survived.

This and other similar cases brought into the hospital started me thinking about the importance of correct protective clothing in survival situations. Once again my thoughts turned to ways of helping to protect aircrew operating in cold environments and the hazards facing downed pilots in Arctic conditions. I stored this up in my mind for the future.

My interest in applied physiology had been stimulated, and as my house jobs were coming to an end I applied for an assistant lecturing post in the Department of Physiology at Glasgow University. Professor Robert Garry was the Regius Professor of Physiology and I knew he was also a member of the Flying Personnel Research Committee (FPRC). I thought he might be able to point me in the right direction for a future career.

GOING FOR A SPIN

After an interview with the Professor and a small selection panel made up of members of staff, I managed to convince them that I was suited to research and lecturing work, and was offered the post of Junior Lecturer in his Department. I took up my new post in the late summer of 1959. In my very first week I had to give a lecture to a hundred or so medical and dental students. Needless to say they were not going to give me an easy ride, and there were many interruptions. Ball bearings came bouncing down steps and bugles were blown. This was baptism by fire – literally, when one of them threw a burning paper aeroplane at me and it landed on the desk. I extinguished the flames as calmly as I could, trying to look as if snuffing out conflagrations was something I did every day. I gave them one or two tips on how to make paper aeroplanes fly better and told them a few amusing examples of failures from my aeromodelling days, to show them I had a sense of humour. As it happened the lecture was on heat exchange physiology – not an easy subject to make interesting - and I turned the interrupted lecture into a discussion (with class interaction) of how important the body's heat exchange system was in flying. You could have heard a pin drop!

That was when I discovered the importance of teaching science that has real practical application. From then on my lectures were slanted towards clinical, aviation and practical and applied working situations. They were well attended and the bugle chants and ball bearings ceased.

It was then that I got in touch with Dr (later Professor) John Durnin. He was a senior member of the Physiology Department who worked from a different building (the old Anderson College) on the campus. I had heard that John was doing some very interesting practical work involving human energy expenditure and oxygen consumption. I asked my Professor if I could join him for a spell, and he agreed.

During the time that followed I was delighted to take part in several very interesting experiments and overjoyed that they all had a practical application. One project I particularly enjoyed was looking at the energy expenditure of people doing all kinds of tasks and work activities; for example, the Theatre Royal in Glasgow was putting on a production of *Coppélia*, and John took the opportunity to measure the energy expended by ballet dancers. He persuaded them to wear bulky backpacks and facemasks during rehearsals one morning. The spectacle of all those ballet dancers strutting around wearing this strange equipment was a sight for sore eyes. It took me all my time to avoid laughing. Nowadays, such a spectacle would quickly be posted on YouTube.

I continued to work with John for some months, and it was he who set me on the road to practical applied physiology. We were a small team and had some marvellous adventures together. I remember climbing Ben Lomond with him, both of us wearing specially adapted full facemasks and bulky backpacks full of complex measuring equipment. When we eventually staggered exhausted to the top, we came face to face with a band of Boy Scouts who had just started to eat their sandwich lunch. When those boys saw us and heard the peculiar hissing noise coming from the valves in the mask they were terrified – they thought we must be invaders from Mars!

With my appetite whetted for applied physiology, I got my next opportunity when I managed to win an ICI Research Fellowship which enabled me to work with a small team of surgeons in the Western Infirmary in Glasgow. They were looking at the clinical possibilities of using oxygen administration at higher atmospheric pressures. Sir Charles Illingworth, Professor of Surgery, had negotiated funding for a very expensive experimental hyperbaric chamber designed to increase oxygen supply to the brain. The idea was to evaluate its use for open-heart surgery, but much to Sir Charles' disgruntlement we diverted it to a very different use; we found that it could be used to great effect in dealing with coal gas poisoning. This was rife in the area at the time as a result of bad housing and rotting pipes and was the cause of much loss of life. The new treatment with hyperbaric oxygen turned out to be a winner, and we saved several patients suffering from accidental coal gas poisoning in this way.

The chamber had been installed in June 1960. Designed to work at double normal atmospheric pressure, it raised the amount of oxygen that could be absorbed into the tissues of the body. Starting with experimental subjects at first, we used it for observing arterial injuries, for example from road traffic accidents or after amputation, or for failed coronary arteries. I remember one poor man being brought in very ill from carbon monoxide poisoning; we literally brought him back from the dead with the aid of the chamber because it cleared the coal gas out of the bloodstream so quickly. We also saved a man's leg from amputation by treating him with hyperbaric oxygen before gangrene could set in.

The efficacy of this wonderful new hyperbaric treatment for these conditions depended on being able to deliver 100% pure oxygen to the patient through a face mask. I was concerned that many of the oxygen face masks currently in use were ill-fitting and leaked air into the mask, dangerously diluting the breathing mixture. I read that a similar problem had been experienced with pilots and aircrew flying at high altitude and that the RAF doctors had got round the problem very cleverly by delivering oxygen to the facemask at a slightly increased pressure (so called 'safety pressure'). In this way any leaks from a badly-fitting mask would be outwards and not inwards and the mixture reaching the pilot therefore would be pure oxygen. I suspected that many of the oxygen masks currently used for a variety of purposes were similarly inefficient and I decided there and then to look into this problem.

I started by referring back to reports of a tragic fire in 1960 aboard a German ship called the *Pagensand* which caught fire in Princes Dock, Glasgow; it was found to have a smouldering cargo of newsprint and other material in the hold. Eight firemen went down into the hold, and in the darkness and fume-filled air seven of them collapsed, and very sadly one man died.

This poor chap had gone down with breathing apparatus to try to get the other men up. In searching the hold he had to squeeze through a narrow opening, and as he was doing so he knocked his nose clip off. He quickly passed out and slumped to the floor. Although his colleagues were working close by, they had no way in the dark of knowing that this man had lost consciousness until it was too late.

I followed this up with a very helpful meeting with the then Chief Firemaster in Glasgow. He allowed me to look at the breathing equipment they were using at that time in their firefighting and rescue operations. I suspected that the mouthpiece and noseclip method of delivering their breathing mixture could in certain unusual circumstances cause problems and recommended that the Fire Brigade might like to consider a more substantial design, perhaps using a whole face mask.

I also discovered during this study that a problem was being encountered by firemen working in dense smoke. If a colleague collapsed, perhaps from inhaling noxious fumes, there was nothing to alert them to what had happened. I suggested it might help if we could devise some form of warning system, so that people would know immediately when a man had lost consciousness. I designed an alarm system which used a pressure sensor in the mouthpiece. When you pass out, your mouth falls open and your jaw goes slack. I reasoned that if this drop in jaw pressure could be detected, it could trigger off a warning sound that could be heard by firefighters working in dark smoke-filled rooms. This was a very simple temporary solution to their problem. With the development of more sophisticated breathing apparatus the need for my device was obviated and I am not sure if it was ever fully adopted.

With my work in pressure chambers I developed an interest in decompression sickness – the problem divers get when they ascend to the surface and the gases in their blood fizz out of solution, like the carbon dioxide gas coming out of a bottle of lemonade. It's a very dangerous condition as the bubbles can get into the brain, with disastrous consequences.

At around this time the Clyde Tunnel was under construction, and to keep the very soft soil of the river bed from caving in on the workers they had to pump air at pressure into the tunnel where the men were working. The police kept picking up men from the streets who appeared to be drunk, but in reality they were suffering from decompression sickness after working in the pressurised tunnel. We had no idea what was causing it, as these men were supposed to spend an hour or so going through a planned decompression schedule after finishing work and before returning to the surface.

We made some enquiries and found that some of these workers were so impatient to get off home or into the pub that they were bypassing this procedure. Some were in so much of a hurry to get back to the outside world that they were even jamming their shovels into the seal of the pressure chamber to release the pressure! After this, signs were put up warning members of the public that if they saw a workman staggering about in the street he might well be dangerously ill, not drunk, and they should call an ambulance.

Although there was no formal health and safety instruction available in those days I tried to persuade the various contractors working on tunnelling operations to make sure their workers were aware of the dangers of taking shortcuts. I believe at least some of them must have heeded the warnings, because for the remainder of my time with the Hyperbaric Unit in Glasgow the number of cases of decompression sickness seemed to decline greatly.

I was now beginning to enjoy my work enormously and felt an inward satisfaction that I was seeing positive results from some of the applied projects I was doing. Yet somewhere in the back of my mind the old interest in flying and applied aviation physiology was beginning to reawaken. I was climbing the first branch of the personal tree of life which Mr McCabe had made me draw, and wondering how long it would be before I could begin to tackle the others.

CHAPTER FOUR

CHAMBER AND CENTRIFUGE

In 1961 something happened which proved to be a turning point in my life; President Kennedy made his famous speech promising the world that the USA would land a man on the Moon by the end of the decade. That was the point at which I began to raise my sights from aviation to space. To enable astronauts to reach the Moon, and hopefully work there, was going to be the greatest challenge man had ever encountered.

There were so many unknowns to explore and so many physiological questions to be answered. I knew immediately that I wanted to be part of the 'space race', as people began to call it. Many people thought Kennedy, who had only just come to power, had made an idle boast and that man could not survive in space, but I had no doubt that his promise would be kept. I couldn't wait.

My interest in space travel had been sparked in 1958 when the Russians sent the first satellite into orbit, and in

April 1961 they had beaten the USA by sending up the first astronaut, Yuri Gagarin. America's response was swift. Although at that stage they had achieved only one manned spaceflight, they were determined to beat the Russians to the Moon. The result was a huge investment in space flight, and I was very keen to play a part in the years to come if I possible could.

I had been greatly inspired by an invitation lecture at Glasgow University given by a visiting professor of aviation physiology, a subject which sounded as if it had been invented just for me. Bill Stewart had helped to found the Institute of Aviation Medicine (IAM) at Farnborough, and was the Commandant at the time. The IAM was successor to the wartime RAF Physiological Laboratory. It had sections investigating all the key aspects of modern flight, such as acceleration, altitude, heat and cold, as well as many other physiological problems facing the aviator. Group Captain Stewart, as he was then, was appointed head in 1946. A former pupil of the Hamilton Academy school, he was promoted to Air Vice-Marshal and awarded a CB and a CBE.

I had to go through a lot of hoops to fulfil my ambition of focusing on aviation medicine. I tried to get a job with Boeing in Seattle, and they expressed interest in taking me on, but at the time I was due to go and see them to discuss matters there was a State Fair and every hotel for miles around was booked solid. Before I could contact them again to make another date, the US aviation Industry was beginning to undergo major changes and I reluctantly had to abandon that route as a way of achieving my dream.

I actually tried to join NASA in the USA, which had only recently been founded (in 1958) and was now switching most of its resources to Kennedy's manned space flight programme. They said they would have considered me for a post, but at that time could not take on non-Americans unless they were members of the armed forces.

In Glasgow, the Professor of Surgery, Sir Charles Illingworth, was pushing for the pressure chamber technique to be applied to surgery, particularly open heart surgery, but that wasn't my interest. I felt it was time to look to new horizons, so I decided to go and see Professor James (later Sir James) Black. He was technically my supervisor during the tenure of the ICI Fellowship and I thought he was just the person to advise me. He had previously established the physiology department at the University of Glasgow, Veterinary College, and had later become an extremely successful pharmacologist. At ICI he developed the drug propranolol, which became the world's best-selling drug; it's a beta blocker, prescribed for anxiety and tension. When he wanted to work on the development of another drug to alleviate stomach ulcers ICI would not fund the work, so he moved to the pharmaceutical company Smith Kline. The result was the development of cimetidine, which overtook propranolol to become the new largest-selling prescription drug, under the name Tagamet. In 1988, with Gertrude Elion and George Hitchings, Sir James went on to win the Nobel Prize in Medicine.

James Black agreed to see me at ICI in Manchester, where he was working at the time. It was a most excellent meeting and he was very supportive. In his own career he had had to fight stiff opposition to his career plans and at times, like me, he had met with discouragement from colleagues. He fully understood the difficult decisions I was having to wrestle with and listened with interest to my thoughts about a career in aviation medicine. He said he thought he might be able to get me to the Institute of Aviation Medicine at Farnborough in a temporary civilian medical attachment.

James Black gave me some words of wisdom which were to guide me throughout my career. 'Never make your current goal your final goal' he said, 'and never let your final goal become your final achievement'. He also told me, 'Don't listen to all the discouraging voices. When you know what you want to do, go balls out and do it.' That was excellent advice, which I did my best to follow.

After my talk with James Black I knew just what I wanted to do and how I could take a major step to achieve it. With the help and contacts of James and Professor Garry I managed to secure the near impossible – a civilian detachment to IAM.

I clearly remember that first arrival at Farnborough in 1961, not least because of an amusing misunderstanding. I was stopped at the gatehouse and asked where I was from, and said I had just come from Ross-shire.

'Russia?' said the rather alarmed young Air Ministry policeman.

'That's right, Ross-shire' I said.

'You've really come from Russia?'

'Yes, Ross-shire, just driven down' I said.

There were frowns and murmurings and I was asked to step into the gatehouse. A few minutes later the younger of the two policemen came over to me and apologised for the delay. 'We've just been on to the adjutant' he said. 'Before we can issue you with a pass he will have to check whether or not you've been vetted.'

I was completely unfamiliar with RAF jargon, much of which had stemmed from fighter pilots during World War 2, and didn't realise that 'being vetted' meant the process of clearing people for security classification. To me, the term was one of a number of euphemisms used in drawing-room conversation to indicate that a domestic pet had been castrated. For one brief but terrifying moment in my confused mind I thought that I might have to undergo a highly personal examination before I could get through the hallowed gates of Farnborough. I know I often told my friends and colleagues that I would give my right arm to get to the Institute of Aviation Medicine, but there were limits to the sacrifices even I would make in order to follow my dream!

It wasn't until Bill Stewart, the Commandant, arrived on the scene that it was all sorted out. Perhaps the chaps on the gate had not heard of Ross-shire, but they had certainly heard of Russia, and with the Cold War at its height they were hardly expecting uninvited guests from beyond the Iron Curtain.

Bill invited me into his office and we discussed the work of the 'lab' and what I might like to do during my time with the Institute. I was so excited that at long last I had reached the home of aviation in Britain and probably the most respected seat of aviation medicine research in the world. Like many thousands of others I had watched television coverage of the Farnborough Air Shows and had marvelled at the displays given by test pilots of all the new aircraft being brought into service with the RAF. I had witnessed the breathtaking flying displays given by the 'V' Bombers, the Avro Vulcan, the Victor and Valiant, and had gasped in disbelief at the thunderous noise (like the tearing of calico cloth) that took the English Electric Lightning soaring to high altitudes in only a few minutes of climb.

I confessed to Bill Stewart that I had a long and burning desire to get involved in the physiology of high-performance flying and to seek ways of protecting the aircrew required to carry it out.

'That's why we are here' said Bill. He explained that with the Cold War at its chilliest, the requirements were for new aircraft that could fly higher, faster and further than anything the Soviets had. The strategy was to fly at altitudes well above the reach of enemy ground-to-air missiles and this potentially placed the aircrew at the limits of physiological endurance, particularly if things went wrong.

'When I take you round the lab you will meet the teams studying the effects on pilots of acceleration, high altitude, climatic problems of heat and cold and many other aspects of this type of tactical flying' explained Bill. 'But first, we must get you fixed up with accommodation.'

He took me over in his staff car to the Officers' Mess. The officers' quarters at Farnborough, where I was to stay, were quite the most anachronistic of buildings you could imagine. They consisted of a series of brick-built bungalows with a long veranda that stretched the full length of the front of the building. They looked so out of place in an establishment dedicated to modern cutting-edge aviation technology. The place was designed exactly like the army messes in India; in fact it was widely believed that the Army Engineers who built the Mess before the First World War had somehow got the plans mixed up and put up a building that should have been destined for Bangalore in India. All that was missing were the 'punkah wallahs' operating the fans to keep the resident officers cool.

The quarters I had been allocated were in the bungalow at the far end of the buildings, and there was a civilian batman who would look after me and another officer. What a rare luxury that turned out to be. I began to feel that perhaps I had missed out when my National Service had been deferred. I consoled myself with the thought that had I been accepted, I might well have ended up fighting in Korea. There was not much luxury and the life there was anything but comfortable. I knew it wouldn't take me long to settle down and enjoy my time at Farnborough, and I was eager to get started.

The following day, as promised, Bill Stewart picked me up in his car and took me on a conducted tour of the Institute. He showed me all the wonderful facilities they had acquired over the years. We went into the large round building which housed the giant man-carrying centrifuge, and we watched the experimental team testing an anti-G suit. They were monitoring heart rate, blood pressure, brain activity and other physiological parameters as an experimental subject was whirled round in a gondola attached to one arm of the centrifuge. It looked horrendous, but Bill assured me the subject was safe in the hands of a highly-experienced monitoring team.

We moved on to the Climatic Research Section, which housed a chamber that could reproduce the different conditions of heat or cold that aircrew might experience. For good measure there was a giant fan which could add to the wind-chill effect of the type to which a downed pilot might be exposed in Arctic conditions.

On that particular morning the experimental team was testing out the efficacy of an air-ventilated suit which had originally been designed at Farnborough. Bill told me that it had started life as a series of plastic pipes sewn into a pair of pyjamas belonging to a senior member of staff, and had been refined and developed into the 'Air Ventilated Garment'. This was routinely used to distribute cooling air over the body surface, keeping aircrew cool when flying in hot conditions.

In an adjacent building another group of investigators were testing life-jackets for buoyancy in a specially designed swimming pool. Bill told me that a new radiant heat chamber was on the cards and in the future this would massively increase their ability to reproduce realistic in-flight thermal conditions. I pricked up my ears at that, and told Bill about my interest in the physiological effects of heat and cold and some of the early experiments I had undertaken in the Physiology Department of Glasgow University. I thought to myself how great it would be to join this team and extend my studies in the direction of aviation.

Bill however had different ideas and told me that he thought they had a place for me working in another Section. He took me over to another building, and there I met Squadron Leader John Ernsting, Head of the High Altitude Research Section, as it was then known. Bill left us to have a chat about the work of the Section and I immediately felt that John was someone I could work with. I instinctively knew that I would benefit from his massive knowledge of aviation medicine and physiology.

JE (as John Ernsting was affectionately known) and his team of doctors, scientists and technical staff were based in the West Wing, a fairly new brick building put up to house a decompression chamber complex in which they proposed to test oxygen systems and other equipment needed to protect aircrew. We discussed the problems facing crew in the event of a sudden and explosive loss of aircraft cabin pressure, and he showed me over the new decompression chamber complex which would soon be used to study the effects of high altitude. It was not fully commissioned yet, but when brought into action it would rival anything NASA had.

Outside the building stood two mobile decompression chambers on trailers, which were being used at the time to test some item of protective equipment. Alongside these was a compression chamber similar to the one I had been using in Glasgow. John told me that he would be delighted if I could join his team and suggested that as a start I might like to use the facilities to extend my studies in hyperbaric medicine. This would be a good lead in to aviation medicine, and I didn't need asking twice to throw in my lot with John and his work. I felt I had arrived where I wanted to be.

Little did I know at the time that John would become not just my mentor and my inspiration but a lifelong friend. Many years later I was best man at his wedding, and he and his wife Joy became very close family friends.

In my first few weeks at the Institute I was desperate to get involved with just about every activity going on there, and I volunteered to be an experimental subject for as many projects as possible. John asked me whether I would be interested in a small but important experimental project which he had been asked to conduct. With a wry smile he explained that it amounted to a study of farting.

'Farting?' I repeated in astonishment.

'Yes, farting' he replied. 'If you accept, you will be testing a pill which contains a detergent designed to break down gas bubbles in the bowel.'

He went on to describe the problem. In modern high-performance aircraft, a rapid climb to altitude could result in any trapped gas in the intestine expanding and causing quite acute abdominal pain. There had been reports from the early Mercury and Gemini astronauts that this could occur in spaceflight and there were fears that flying performance in space and in conventional flight might be compromised. I jumped at the chance to participate, but laughed to myself that my very first involvement in aerospace medicine should be so alimentary.

The experiment involved several of us who were living in the Officers' Mess at the time. We were required to eat two tins of Heinz curried baked beans the previous evening and avoid emptying our bowels the following morning. We then went into the decompression chamber and ascended to a simulated altitude. Each of us recorded on a line chart an estimate of how much abdominal pain we had experienced during the ascent. One group was given the pill, one a placebo. You can imagine how unpleasant the atmosphere was by the end of the experiment!

One day when we were doing this, our toilet in the West Wing was out of order. I was desperate to 'go' at the end of the experiment and set out on a frantic hundred-yard dash to the nearest convenience in the HQ building. Just as I reached the door the Commandant stopped me and languidly started asking how I was getting on. He obviously had all the time in the world, but I was seconds from disaster. I made it, but it was touch and go.

It was quite disappointing to discover later that all our discomfort had been in vain. There was no experimental evidence whatsoever that the pill did what it claimed for aircrew and our suggestion for an alternative approach to the problem - avoiding certain gas-producing foods - was, I believe, finally taken up by NASA in the Apollo astronaut training programme. As for me, I will never be able to look a curried baked bean in the face again!

It wasn't long before I was given my own office/laboratory on the upper floor of the West Wing. That was when I first met the legendary Flight Lieutenant John Billingham, and it happened in the most extraordinary way. On the first day in my new office I was sitting at my desk reading some papers when I heard a tapping coming from a strange metallic tower sitting in the corner. It appeared to have been constructed from two large oil drums with an access ladder fixed to the front of the contraption. I assumed that this had been a piece of apparatus used in some experiment and left by the previous occupant of the laboratory.

Once again the tapping noise emanated from the tower, this time a bit louder, and I took a few steps up the ladder and peered into oil drum to see if I could find the source of the noise.

It was full of water. To my astonishment a head appeared above the water, a mouthpiece was removed and a voice exclaimed 'Good morning, I wonder if you would be so kind as to change over my breathing mixture by turning on the green tap'. It was John Billingham, carrying out an off-the-wall experiment as usual. Although I never discovered exactly what he was doing in the oil drums, I suspect it was something to do with the United States Space Programme, for he later became Head of Life Sciences for NASA.

John Billingham was a talented and highly dedicated man who made his name some time before my arrival at the 'lab'.

He took on an experiment in desert survival and demonstrated that a downed pilot could stay alive until rescued by drinking nothing but the juice of crushed snails. These white snails were found in abundance in the Libyan desert and John proved that the juice extracted from them, disgusting as it must have tasted, could provide a valuable source of water for desert survivors. No one else would undertake such an unpleasant experiment, but John was game. He suffered no more than some slight nausea and, I understand from his colleagues, foul-smelling breath. I was greatly impressed by the dedication of this officer, and there seemed to be many other like-minded and dedicated staff in every Section of the Institute.

John Ernsting was interested in the work I had been doing in Glasgow with the Hyperbaric Unit, and was very supportive in helping me to plan out experiments that I could usefully carry out in the small pressure chamber. He brought together a team of technicians and RAF NCOs who were happy to assist me in the various projects we were to conduct over the next few months. He also gave me the services of a temporary laboratory technician who would help me to analyse the results my experiments. This new and very welcome arrival to my little team was Beatrice Bickerton. She was a delightful girl with a wicked sense of humour. She brought a lovely feminine touch to the mainly male-dominated team of doctors, scientists and technicians that made up the staff of the Institute.

Beatrice seemed fascinated by my Scottish accent and used to sing snatches of singer Andy Stewart's well-known songs. She would sometimes greet me in the morning with the words from Andy's famous song, *Donald where's yer troosers?* and burst out laughing at my reaction.

'I love the way you Scottish men roll your arse' I thought she said one day as we were analysing results of the latest experiment. Seeing the puzzled look on my face she went on, 'No I'm not talking about your ARSE, the way you Scots pronounce your 'Rs'. We both collapsed in mirth. After that she was always trying to get me to say '*Hoch aye the noo, we'll hae a wee blow at the pipes*'.

Quite strange I thought, as I believed I had a neutral accent and certainly didn't think of myself as a typical 'Rob Roy'. But I enjoyed her company so much that I really didn't mind her poking a little fun at me.

What a talented girl Beatrice turned out to be. I became very fond of her, although I knew I was not in with a snowball's chance in hell of dating her. She was a very attractive girl, a qualified pilot and flying instructor, and she was very popular with the test pilots who were in abundance around Farnborough. Although she never let on to anyone, her father owned Denham Airfield and I believe, half the old Denham film studios. She invited me on a few occasions to have Sunday lunch and meet her parents in Denham. She lived in a quite magnificent house close to Denham Airfield and when I met her father, Dr Myles Bickerton. I found him to be a very pleasant and highly intelligent man. He was a retired ophthalmic surgeon and we had most interesting discussions about the importance of vision in flying. He took me to one of the buildings that formed part of the old film studio complex and proudly showed me his somewhat unusual collection of earth-moving vehicles. They looked just like giant Tonka Toys, and he loved every one of them.

Best of all, on these visits to Denham, Beatrice taught me to fly in her own aeroplane, a Miles Gemini. It was a twin-engine light aircraft, not particularly easy to handle and not really suitable as a first training aircraft, but I took to flying like a duck to water and before long had fully mastered the controls. My longing to fly was at last beginning to be satisfied, and I was grateful to Beatrice for making that happen. Already my detachment to RAF Farnborough had brought me in touch with test pilots and an overwhelming variety of military and civilian aircraft, and I felt my dreams might just be coming true. I wondered where and when the next opportunity to fly might come.

I was well aware that as a civilian my participation in the work of IAM was limited for the moment to projects that were not of a highly security sensitive nature. I longed for my security clearance to a higher classification to come through and allow me to take a more active part in the Section's activities. John Ernsting understood my frustration and assured me that it wouldn't be long, but in the meantime he asked me to join him in an experiment he had been longing to do for some time. It was a profound hypoxia experiment which arose from a paper John had read in a medical journal, in which a group of clinicians had come up with an idea for treating cancer; if you could deplete the oxygen in all the cancer cells and then flash-irradiate them, they believed you would get much more effective killing of tumour tissue.

He was quite up front about the fact that it was dangerous, and said he would do it first. As I watched, he took two breaths of pure nitrogen to sink his oxygen level down as close to zero as possible. The measuring instruments registered an alarming fall in tissue oxygen and the brain waves were beginning to show worrying changes. At the point when I considered it dangerous to continue I restored the pure oxygen supply and John came round almost immediately. He was unscathed by the experience, although I was shaking like a leaf at the responsibility and total reliance on my judgement that John had placed on me.

This sort of experiment is possible only because the brain has a rather surprising response to an intake of pure nitrogen. As long as it detects normal-pressure inhalation and normal CO_2 exhalation, it thinks everything's going fine. No panic sets in, and the person breathing the nitrogen simply keels peacefully over and dies shortly afterwards of suffocation, unless resuscitated very quickly. Just such an accident knocked out five technicians on NASA's Columbia programme in 1981, two of them dying before they could be revived.

Despite John's reluctance to let me act as subject, he eventually relented and we swapped places. I have no recollection of events during the experiment, although John assured me that I was only out for ten or fifteen seconds. What amazed me most was that during that brief time I had the longest, most protracted and vivid dream - it felt like months. I now understood why they say a drowning man sees his life flash before him. I can well believe it.

Although that rather terrifying experiment showed that it was possible to drop tissue oxygen levels to very low values, it was considered too dangerous and unpredictable to be adopted as a clinical treatment. But that experience, and my willingness to participate in such a dangerous experiment, created a strong and lasting bond between John Ernsting and myself. It also showed me that the Institute, busy as it was, could still find time to carry out experiments and investigations that were not strictly for military operations but could be used for clinical purposes, ultimately to help mankind. I noted and admired this attitude and quietly stored up the idea for the future.

John really was an amazing fellow and I was extremely impressed by him and remained so. One of the things he taught me was the importance of accuracy in every project and every experiment, pointing out that a life might depend on it. As a team leader he was very strict and demanding, but he was enormously respected by everyone in the Institute. His word was law.

That wonderful team spirit John engendered reflected the fact that we were all working with a single aim; to improve the safety and comfort of aircrew in flight. No one in the Institute at that time seemed to be trying to promote their own interests, and there was none of this nonsense I'm afraid we get in much of the medical profession of 'publish or perish', or to have the letters 'BTA' (Been To America) metaphorically after your name. Most of the people working at the lab were highly qualified men, some of whom had had to do National Service, and I couldn't help but admire the 'esprit de corps' they lived by.

At long last my security clearance came through, and this enabled me to take part in more of the militarily-orientated test projects. John asked me to join forces with Flight Lieutenant Pete Wagner, who was testing the efficacy of new protective assemblies which had been developed for very high altitude flying in strategic operational roles. Although the aircraft were operating at heights well above the range of enemy surface-to-air missiles, there was always a danger of sudden explosive loss of cabin pressure. This is where the protective assemblies and oxygen delivery systems would come in to keep the pilot conscious for enough time to bring the aircraft down to safer altitudes.

Day after day we would don various pieces of experimental protective equipment and assemblies and 'test fly' them in the decompression chamber, simulating explosive loss of cabin pressure. To begin with it was quite nerve-racking, but I was always confident that Pete and his team of highly-trained technicians would look after me if I needed to be brought down in a 'crash descent' to ground level. Fortunately this was only rarely needed and I got quite used to these experiments as time went on.

There were occasions when the protective assemblies and ourselves as subjects were tested to limits, and these remained a slight source of anxiety to me. My security classification did not allow me to know the final altitude the chamber would reach with the rapid decompression. That was highly confidential and was treated on a strictly need-to-know basis. Although Peter understood the 'butterflies in the stomach' feeling which every experimental subject has when facing the unexpected and unknown, he was not allowed to divulge the final operating altitude we would reach in the chamber. The first time I asked him what altitude profile we were using that day, he replied 'we are going to heights, Gordon, where angels fear to tread', adding with a reassuring smile 'but then angels don't have the protective assemblies that we do!' After that, whenever he mentioned that it was an 'angel day' that cryptic message was all I needed to prepare myself for the experiment, and all my anxieties seemed to evaporate quickly.

Sometimes the equipment we were testing included a partial pressure helmet, which made us all look like budding astronauts. The thought that the astronauts and ourselves shared some of the kit pleased me no end, and I began to relax and actually enjoy the experience.

The experiments which John Ernsting and the team carried out were not always quite so dangerous, and sometimes they turned out to be a great source of amusement to our colleagues. In one of our test projects, we were required to measure brain activity at very high altitude. To get over some recording difficulties we needed to shave several patches the size of an old penny on our scalps and sew in stainless steel sutures to act as recording electrodes. It wasn't exactly a comfortable experience, but conventional electrodes were quite useless during high altitude decompressions and we had no alternative. For the same reason we had to record the activity of the heart by using home-made electrodes fashioned from a kitchen nutmeg grater. The sharp points punctured the surface of the skin, and after a long period of wear they became quite painful and irritating.

One day the Commandant phoned to invite a few members of the Institute who were working on high-altitude protection to lunch with one of the visiting top brass in the RAF. He very kindly included me in the luncheon party. John hurriedly changed into uniform and I into my suit, but he insisted that we could not take the sutures out until the experiment was over. We had to sit there in the dining room of the Officers' Mess making polite conversation with these strange wires sticking out of our heads. The other members of the Mess stared at us in disbelief, and I am certain that the senior officer must have thought we were very odd people indeed. Such were the penalties of working at the Institute, but I wouldn't have missed the opportunity for anything.

As my time at the Institute went on I took every available opportunity to become involved with the experiments and investigations being conducted in other sections of the lab. There was so much going on that I couldn't hope to cover more than a fraction of the activities. As I gained more experience I became more and more convinced that I was on the right lines and destined for a career in aviation medicine. I even managed to extend my experiences to the Empire Test Pilots' School (ETPS), which at that time was located at Farnborough. There was no possibility whatsoever of flying with them, but their classroom and ground training accommodation was next door to the IAM and I would sometimes join the test pilots in the bar of their Mess. It was rarely packed, as these pilots spent the day test flying various aircraft types and most evenings in deep study within their rooms. A few of them, however, enjoyed the different and more relaxed atmosphere of our No 1 Mess and would sometimes join us in our bar for a change of scene.

It was then that I got to know one of these ETPS test pilots well. One balmy summer evening I went out for a stroll with him in the Mess garden. We talked about the work of a test pilot, comparing and contrasting it with the work being carried out at the Institute. We agreed that there were some similarities between the two roles. He expressed amazement that as a test pilot he was required to know every tiny detail of every system and subsystem of a new aircraft, yet he was given little information about the most important system in test flying – the human body, and the mind of the pilot.

This was a very interesting observation, which seemed to highlight a gap in communication between the aircrew at the 'sharp end' and the doctors and scientists carrying out aviation medical research and development at the Institute. I resolved there and then that if I was ever in a position to correct this I would do so, and tucked the thought into the back of my mind for the future.

Our walk continued down the Mess garden and towards the perimeter fence of the airfield. We looked up to see high in the heavens a reproduction SE5A biplane flying over, a First World War fighter. It left a wonderful aroma of burnt castor oil in its wake. I gather it had been built by apprentices of the Royal Aircraft Establishment (RAE), and only the Station Commander at RAF Farnborough was allowed to fly it. My test pilot friend commented on this evocative scene and told me he gained inspiration from being close to the place where Colonel Samuel Franklin Cody (1867-1913) had worked on the design and development of his flying machines. He regarded Cody as the first British 'test pilot' and pointed to the very spot, only a few yards from where we were standing, where the Colonel had taken off in the flimsy biplane which he had designed and built himself.

With that flight on 16th October 1908, Cody became the first man in Britain to achieve powered flight. Although he flew for just 27 seconds and covered a distance of only 1390ft at a height of 30ft, it was a truly remarkable achievement of its day, and many pilots to follow, including present-day test pilots, drew great inspiration from his magnificent efforts.

When we reached the end of the Mess garden, my friend pointed to 'Cody's Tree', the monument to the Colonel's achievement all these years ago. It was the remains of the beech tree Cody had used to tether his aeroplane in order to measure the thrust of his aero engines at maximum revolutions. Now black and leafless and mostly preserved with a patchwork of resin and glass fibre, it occupied a grass strip in front of the famous 'Black Sheds' which Cody had used in his early pioneering days. It stood proudly on its stone plinth, reminding us of the early history of the Royal Aircraft Establishment.

Cody had battled to prove his theories about flight in the face of a mountain of opposition before he was finally recognised by being commissioned to develop man-carrying kites and gliders for military use. I admired the qualities of passion, perseverance and persuasion which had driven him on to achieve his final goal. These were qualities which I would need to emulate if I too wanted to achieve my dreams of a career in aerospace medicine.

That tree had an additional significance. As soon as I saw it I was reminded of something; the tree of life which I had been instructed to draw by the wonderful Mr McCabe all those years earlier. Cody's tree became an inspiration to me, and I would return to it many times over the years that followed.

As the time approached for me to leave IAM and return to Scotland, I went to see Bill Stewart and asked him if there was a possibility that he might find me a permanent post so that I could carry on my work at Farnborough. His answer came as quite a blow. They were not able at the time to take on any more than the present complement of staff, and for the immediate future any replacements would be from serving officers rather than civilians. He said the only way for me to carry on working at the IAM would be to join the RAF, but he warned me that the competition for jobs was fierce, with the cream of the university graduates applying. He couldn't make any promises, but he assured me he would do what he could. I knew Bill Stewart was a man of his word, and I felt he would move Heaven and Earth to help me in my career.

I went back to my parents' place in Fortrose in Ross-shire and whiled away a few days ambling along the seashore and mowing the grass, mulling over what I should do next. In the end I decided to take the gamble and put in an application to the medical branch of the RAF. I phoned them in Tavistock Square, and they invited me for interview in two days' time.

When the day came I was interviewed by a chap called Group Captain Sandow, who was quite a character. After a brief preliminary chat he made a phone call and sent me over to Holborn for a medical, which went fine, to my relief; they said I had slight visual astigmatism, but that was nothing to worry about as I was not planning to be a fighter pilot. Group Captain Sandow said that if I was 'mad enough to join the mob' they would be happy to have me. I would be granted a three-year short service commission as Medical Officer with the rank of Flight Lieutenant.

I felt glad that I had made such a life-changing decision and set about the paperwork needed for my resignation from the ICI Research Fellowship. I took that opportunity to say how much I had enjoyed my time with the surgical team, and thanked Dr Black for all his help and encouragement. I was now looking forward to becoming an RAF officer. I thought I would then be able to walk straight into the job I wanted at Farnborough and carry on the work I had been doing with John Ernsting and the team. Unfortunately I had another think coming.

In due course, an official-looking letter arrived on my doorstep telling me to report for basic training in the Medical Training Establishment at RAF Freckleton in Lancashire.

First I had to attend a formal (and I hoped final) interview at RAF Biggin Hill so that senior RAF officers could look me over and make sure I was officer material. The interview was short and rather irrelevant, I thought. It boiled down to finding out which books and newspapers I read and why I wanted to join the Service. My answers seemed to satisfy them, and I was informed that I had officially been accepted into the RAF.

I was walking on air. I was still a long way off achieving my goal of joining the space race, but it was a good start and I couldn't wait to begin a new phase of my life and career.

CHAPTER FIVE

DESERT BOOTS AND FLYING SUITS

My two weeks' basic training at RAF Freckleton did not get off to an auspicious start. The chap who welcomed me on the gate explained to me that contrary to what I had been told so far, I had not really joined the RAF. 'Turn your car round and go right back!' he told me.

I was mystified, until it was later explained to me that this man's self-appointed mission in life was to stop other young doctors joining the Air Force out of sheer jealousy. I think he had become marooned in a transient families' unit and harboured some resentment.

I soon learned the peculiarities of RAF etiquette; everything from who to salute to the correct procedure for passing round the port decanter at a formal dining–in night. We were given the opportunity to put much of what we had learned into practice. They arranged a dining-in night in the Officers' Mess for us. I'm glad to say the port decanter was passed correctly and nobody had to pay the penalty of buying a round of drinks for everybody present at the table.

Unfortunately too much of it, and other wines and spirits, was consumed, and the evening descended into complete chaos. Members of the course, quite tipsy by then, tried to move the static Spitfire at the entrance gate. This was nothing new; countless other course members had done the same thing after formal dinner evenings. In the past the police had had to intervene when a previous entrant Medical Officer pushed the Spitfire out onto the main road, blocking traffic for a considerable time while engineers and technicians attempted a retrieval. One can only imagine what the motorist who reported the incident felt when he spotted a WW2 fighter apparently landing or taking off from a main road.

As a result of this performance, the wheels of the aeroplane were chained down to the concrete base, so there was no hope of repeating that prank. Not to be outdone, one of our group managed to force entry into the aeroplane and sit in the cockpit, and we all took turns at playing at being a Spitfire pilot. It was a silly and childish experience, if a memorable one, and one I paid for dearly, because years of dust and oil in the cockpit nearly ruined my Mess dress uniform. Fortunately the cleaners managed to restore it to its original condition.

Parade drill was a bit of a waste of time, and realising this, we new boys took great pleasure in halting when the drill sergeant told us to go on, turning right when he said left and turning left when he said right. The uniform fitting was quite a training exercise in itself, and I soon found, literally to my cost, just how much the military tailor Gieves charged for a new uniform.

Finally our postings were read out, and I waited for confirmation that I would soon be on my way back to Farnborough. I had not yet learned that the Forces don't work quite like that. The powers that be would decide where they were going to send me, and it certainly wouldn't be an immediate posting back to Farnborough, at least not yet.

I was shocked to be told that I was to be posted to Bahrain, in the Persian Gulf, for the full three-year tour. I must confess that at that time I had never even heard of Bahrain. I assumed someone had made a silly mistake, so I contacted the Medical Branch Headquarters up in London. They were very helpful and understanding of the situation and explained that there was an unwritten rule that new doctors coming in to the Medical Branch never started by joining a specialised unit. Bahrain it would have to be. I consoled myself with the thought that the pathway to the Institute might be tortuous, but it was still open.

I was leaving a rather nice little sports car behind, a Triumph TR2, and had to ask my father to sell it for me as there was no point in leaving it to go rusty for three years. More of my passion for cars later.

Before I took up my posting I had to endure a series of inoculations, which turned out to be very painful and to make me briefly feel very ill. Yellow fever, cholera, typhoid – everything you could think of was stabbed into my arm. By the time they had finished I felt dizzy and seemed to be floating two feet off the ground. Fortunately we were allowed 24 hours off duty to get over the effects, and I could see why.

A spell at RAF Halton taught us how to deal with our overseas posting and how to avoid catching tropical diseases and escape food poisoning. It was there that I learned that my job would be very similar to that of a GP back home, looking after servicemen and their families –very different from the academic and research work I was used to, but I was sure I could make the most of it and turn it into an interesting and valuable experience.

Once I was fully indoctrinated into the ways of Service life, it was time for me to take up my posting to the Middle East. First I would spend some time in the Port of Aden on the Red Sea, where there was a strong military presence. The headquarters of RAF Middle East Command was based there and the top brass of the Medical Branch had planned that I should first spend some time at RAF Khormaksar and the associated Military Hospitals in the area. The badge portrayed an Arab dhow and the motto was 'into the remote places'. Remote it certainly was, but the top brass considered it essential as a way of easing me into the unfamiliar life and work of a Medical Officer before taking up my destination posting to RAF Muharraq in Bahrain.

How right they were. Even before we took off from the UK on a chartered troop carrier aircraft bound for Aden, I began to notice several strange and unfamiliar ways in which the RAF did things. First of all we were picked up in a coach which had, of all things, rear-facing seats. It turned out to be quite a strange experience travelling through the roads and streets leading to the airport with everybody facing the wrong way. This was clearly an introduction to some of the peculiar Service ways, and it was not confined to the RAF.

I had heard that the Royal Navy pretended that the grass on their Land Based Fleet Air Arm Stations was the sea, and anyone who dared to step on to the forbidden area was rushed to the Sick Bay to pay the penalty of immediate hosing down with fresh water, just as they would be treated at sea. The RAF had not gone quite as far as that, but in this case they had followed the Navy example of getting personnel used to the ways of the Service by treating passengers in every form of transport, including buses, as if they were airborne. I couldn't complain, as my colleagues at Farnborough had recommended rear-facing seats as a safety measure in the event of a crash landing. Many of their experiments which I had recently witnessed at the Institute confirmed that rearward-facing seats could help to prevent serious or life-threatening injury. Although the RAF had taken up their advice, they never managed to persuade the airlines to follow their example.

The flight out to Aden was long but reasonably comfortable. Once again I was reminded that I was now in the Service when the in-flight lunch turned out to be a cardboard box containing a cellophane packet of biscuits, an unripe green apple and a packet of chewing gum. I was learning fast, and there were more strange examples of Service life to come.

When we landed at the airfield at Aden and started to disembark from the aeroplane I was met by a blast of hot air which I thought at first must be coming from the aircraft engines. Not a bit of it - this was my first encounter with the climate of the Middle East, and boy was it overpowering. It was just like being in a sauna, and the lightweight suit I had chosen to travel in (we never travelled in uniform) became soaked in perspiration even before I reached the terminal building. What a welcome, I thought. I began to wonder what on earth I was doing there. Then I remembered the old Service expression 'if you can't stand the heat get out of the kitchen'. How appropriate, I thought. I decided there and then that whatever I came up against I would make the most of my situation and enjoy this posting and the new experiences it had to offer.

I was met by the Senior Medical Officer and taken in his Land Rover to the Red Sea Hotel, an RAF transit hotel. How it had ever been dignified by the name 'hotel' I will never know. Perhaps I was expecting my first night in the Middle East to be in a lovely air-conditioned swish establishment like the famous Raffles Hotel in Singapore. My expectations were suddenly and completely shattered. Even after all these years it is still the ghastliest place I've ever stayed in. The room looked straight over to the sea wall, where I watched a procession of Arabs walk up to answer the call of nature. It was nothing more than an open-air communal latrine. The Red Sea Hotel had been built next to a goat market, and the awful smell that wafted in to the rooms, coupled with the inevitable swarms of flies, added to the general unpleasantness of the place.

I had another shock when I unpacked the clothes that Gieves had supplied. The khaki drill they had given me must have been in stock for the best part of a century. They had given me shorts, socks, shirt, epaulettes – it made me look like an overgrown boy scout. I don't think my fellow officers resident in the hotel had ever seen anything quite like it before. Everyone was looking at me as if I was from another planet, or another age.

'Where the hell did you get that?' one of my colleagues exclaimed between snorts of derisive laughter. He said it would have been far better to have waited and had some kit made out there. If only I had known. He whisked me off to a tailor, who made me up a complete set of uniform pretty much on the spot, for a very reasonable price.

I didn't have to put up with the Red Sea Hotel for very long, as I was transferred to the RAF Khormaksar Officers' Mess. It was total luxury compared with the transit accommodation I had recently endured and I began to enjoy myself and relish my new life in the Service.

It is strange that wherever you go in the world you seem to meet someone you know. One evening I met Marjorie 'Midge' Langmuir in the bar of the Officers' Mess. She had been in my class all the way through Medical School in Glasgow and had been a fellow house doctor during my time in the old Raigmore Hospital in Inverness. It was wonderful to meet up with her again, and we had a long chat in the bar reminiscing about the old days.

Marjorie was working as a doctor with British Petroleum (BP) in the refinery at Little Aden, but she was a regular visitor to the RAF Station and joined in the social life of the base. She gave me very good advice about where to go and what to see around Aden, and advised me what were good bargains and purchases to be had in the Crescent shopping area of the old town. More importantly, she warned me where it was not safe to go, and related tales of British troops who in the past had wandered into territory which was strictly out of bounds. They had reportedly suffered dreadful consequences at the hands of the rebels who dwelt there. I took note of her good advice.

In the weeks before taking up my posting in Bahrain, I continued to gain experience of working in the hospital at Steamer Point and in the Medical Centre on the RAF station. It was while I was standing in for one of the doctors in the

Medical Centre that I had a second and even stranger reunion with a colleague from the past. I had just started to take the morning sick parade when the corporal medic came into my consulting room and asked if I could see some people who had arrived unexpectedly at the Centre. I was confronted by three men dressed in Arab costume sitting in the waiting area. The corporal said they were from a mission hospital in the wilds of the Radfan Mountain area and made regular annual visits to the Medical Centre to seek supplies.

I quietly asked the corporal if any of them could speak English. One of the three men spoke up.

'Yes I do' he said, 'and if I'm not very much mistaken, you are Gordon Sharp.'

To my astonishment he turned out to be a student who had been a year or so ahead of me at medical school in Glasgow.

'What on earth are you doing here?' I blurted out, desperately trying to remember his name.

'I'm afraid that I am begging, Gordon' he said, showing me a rubber breathing bag from an antiquated anaesthetic machine. 'We are badly needing a replacement.'

I had to agree. The bag was in a dreadful state, badly perished, and where the rubber had torn it had been patched up with sticking plasters. It was not only useless but potentially dangerous.

'The Mission Hospital is very short of funds and medical supplies' he explained. 'We are eternally grateful for any help we can get from the RAF to keep us going.'

I remembered this chap only as Brian - I never got to know his surname. He was a rather shy individual who tended to keep his own company and could sometimes be seen chatting with the Divinity students. I had met him from time to time in the lunch hall of the Men's Union at Glasgow University, but I hadn't really got to know him all that well. I was surprised that he remembered who I was.

The Corporal interrupted at this point to explain that this was an annual occurrence and the Medical Centre had been given permission by HQ Middle East Command to supply the Mission Hospital with any medicines, dressings, instruments and anything else which was surplus to requirements.

'We have always managed to find something which is surplus to our needs' said the Corporal with a knowing look, 'and with your permission, sir, we could do so now.'

'Of course! I replied. 'Give them whatever you can find.'

With that, the corporal and the other two men went through to the dispensary storeroom. They emerged later with several bags packed to the gunwales with I know not what, but I gathered from the broad grin on the faces of the two men that their visit had been very fruitful.

Time was desperately short, and I wanted to hear all about Brian's work and how he had come to be involved with the Church and its Mission Hospital in the wilds of Aden, but I had to get back to my busy clinic, and he had to set off early on a long, hot and tiring journey back to his mission in the Radfan Mountains. There was only time to bid each other a brief farewell, but his thanks and appreciation of the supplies we had provided were quite humbling. I returned to my duties with a feeling that I had done my good deed for the day. I never saw or heard from Brian again and have often wondered what became of him, his mission and the hospital.

My short time in Aden was beginning to run out, and I

was now due to take up my main posting in Bahrain. I had not yet fully acclimatised to the unrelenting heat of the desert. I still found it unbearable at times and wasn't too sorry when my posting notice eventually came through for a transfer to Bahrain in the Persian Gulf.

I was given a few days' leave to pack up my things ready for the flight and took the opportunity to relax and join some of the officers going to the Golden Beach. But I still hadn't learned my lesson and strode out on to the beautiful golden sands without the protection of a pair of flip-flops on my feet. (My instructor at RAF Halton would have had a fit - it was a cardinal rule always to have something on your feet). It was like walking on a stove. My feet were quite badly burned and began to swell up.

That night in the Mess I joined my friends for farewell drinks. At one point I felt distinctly light-headed and thought I would pass out, but I stuck with it, not wanting to let the medical profession down by letting them think I couldn't hold my drink. I staggered through the evening somehow and eventually made it to bed. As the RAF pilots would say 'I climbed to an altitude of two feet, levelled out and crashed out.' I still had lots to learn about coping with desert conditions.

After the infernal heat of Aden it was a relief to get on to the aircraft and head for what I had been told was the much less trying climate of RAF Muharraq in Bahrain.

Muharraq was quite lush by comparison with Aden, and there were lots of date palms lining the roadways. There seemed to be plenty of grass around and I was quite impressed with the Officers' Mess, which was set in a pleasant garden full of bougainvillea trees with a strip of grass that ran down to the beach. The lawns and bushes seemed to be watered at frequent intervals to keep them nicely green and lush. Bahrain benefited from a huge artesian well deep down below the desert so there was no shortage of water there.

However, I soon discovered a snag to this 'green and pleasant land'. The smell of sewage was quite unpleasant and my accommodation block – a bungalow-type building - stood at the end of a long sewage pipe which projected out into the sea. This had been an adequate arrangement when Bahrain had been built, but the population had grown enormously since the Kuwait crisis when several squadrons were deployed to the station. There was practically no tidal movement, so the sewage effluent just stayed where it was and gently sloshed in and out and on to the sandy strip of shore below my bedroom window. We used to call the little spit where the pipe ran out Turd Point.

Every now and then entertainers came out to put on a show for us, and on one occasion I was asked to make the arrangements for a visit by the singer Dickie Valentine, who was then quite a big name back in Britain. He arrived with a troupe of chorus girls and hangers-on. The morning after his arrival I looked out of my window to see Dickie, dressed in a pair of bright red trunks, charging straight down Turd Point. I was horrified. I tried to run out to stop him, but it was too late. He must have got a terrible shock when he dived into that blue sea and realised that most of it wasn't sea at all.

We pointed him in the direction of the shower block and I'm pleased to say that he did see the funny side, but the Entertainments Officer wasn't very pleased at all by our lapse of hospitality. We took greater care of that from then on.

The comedian Tommy Cooper was another star from the

UK who came to put on a show for us. The lighting was always breaking down, and it managed to do so right in the middle of his act. Tommy ordered us to start clapping, and as soon as we did so, the lights came on again. 'There you are, you see' he said. 'Many hands make light work.' I never could decide whether he had arranged for the lights to go out or if he simply had a funny routine ready for every occasion.

Not long after my arrival I was briefed by my Senior Medical Officer, Wing Commander Ian Mercer, on the type of work I would be involved in for the duration of my three-year tour in Bahrain. I was going to be a member of a medical team that consisted of three other flight lieutenant Medical Officers, a Squadron Leader MO and the Wing Commander. As the most recent arrival to the Medical Team, I was replacing a doctor who had come to the end of his tour and had returned to the UK. I was put in charge of the Hospital Section of the Station Medical Centre. Like the rest of the medical facilities on the station, the hospital part was a leftover from the days of the Kuwait operation when RAF Bahrain had found itself at the centre of military operations in the Middle East. Now redundant and decommissioned, the small hospital had been absorbed into the Medical Centre and was being used as a holding ward for patients being transferred to the main RAF hospitals in Aden. It was also being used for acute admissions and was well-equipped, with a large ward, an officers' ward, offices, consulting rooms, X-ray facilities and even a disused operating theatre. We had a team of Princess Mary's RAF Nursing Officers and NCOs and men of the Medical Branch who assisted in the running of the medical complex. It was just like being in charge of my very own hospital, and I enjoyed the relative freedom of being able to take control my own working schedule. It was a unique position and responsibility for a junior medical officer and it came to my rescue when a few nagging doubts began to enter my head.

Although I was beginning to enjoy the novelty of my new work and life in the RAF, there were moments when I began to question whether I had taken the right course of action by joining the Service. Had I taken the wrong career pathway and destroyed my chances of getting back into research and development work, as I longed to do? Bill Stewart had been very supportive and had promised me he would do everything in his power to help. John Ernsting too had said he hoped he would soon be welcoming me back to IAM. But in the Service, things were liable to change rapidly, and my future plans were always at risk of being shattered by what the RAF called 'the exigencies of the Service'. I had a few sleepless nights worrying that I might end up like the frustrated and bitter Medical Officer who had tried to turn me back at the Station gate on my first day at RAF Freckleton.

It was then that my thoughts turned to previous visits I had made to Cody's Tree. I had studied more of Cody's life and work and knew he too had suffered many of the discouraging setbacks that were now occasionally nagging at me. I recalled that his dreams of developing military flying machines had turned out to be a bumpy ride for him. The military were not convinced about investing in new flimsy aeroplanes that were prone to crashing, and withdrew their funding for his project. He was forced to continue his experiments and flight trials using his own funds and working in a shed at Laffans Plain near Farnborough with a tiny team of helpers and volunteers. His perseverance paid off, and as we know he went on to do great things in the aviation world.

Cody's example gave me the inspiration to press on with my interests in aviation physiology and medicine. I believed that if he could make giant strides on a shoestring with bags of passion and enthusiasm, then so could I. There was no way I could match up to the marvellous work coming out of IAM Farnborough, but I could try and do some kind of field research work here in Bahrain. If nothing else it would preserve my sanity.

But how and where I could scrape together even the basic equipment needed to get me started? I had no idea, until something of a minor miracle happened, which boosted my morale and changed everything. I was probing around in the disused theatre of the old hospital when I discovered a treasure trove of redundant equipment, including anaesthetic machines, clinical measuring equipment and all manner of other bits and bobs. It even had an X-ray suite which was in good working order, which we used for diagnosing suspected bone fractures. Here was the answer to my prayers. To an inveterate gadget man and inventor like me it was a gift from the gods, and it was not long before I was indulging my love of experimentation and medical detective work again.

The first little mystery I was called upon to solve involved members of the Hunter squadron who kept coming in complaining of severe back pain. One or two even had to be hospitalised with it. The Squadron Commander was mystified, as he said nothing had changed to account for this sudden onset of back trouble. I set to work to solve the problem and used the little trick I had learned from my time in Glasgow - to look at every action involved in the operational task. As part of this I carefully observed the pilots getting in and out of the aircraft. They were tall blokes and when they sat on the ejector seat and tried to close the canopy I noticed that they had to duck their heads and loosen their safety harnesses. Not only was this an uncomfortable position for flying, but if they had to eject from a stricken aircraft they would almost certainly have injured their spines. This unacceptable sitting position was the obvious cause of the back problems. But why hadn't it been happening before?

I made some investigations and discovered that the seat they were sitting on contained all the survival kit. Because they were flying in desert areas, extra water containers had been put in; they were only the size of cigarette packets, but there were dozens of them. This raised the height of the seat pack and accordingly the pilot's sitting height. I wrote to John Ernsting to ask his advice and through his good offices we managed to get the parachute packers to redistribute the water containers and get the seat down. Result – no more back pain.

One day we had a serious incident to deal with. We received a message that an aircraft had crashed in the Muscat region and an RAF pilot attached to the Sultan of Oman's air force, a man I knew, had been badly injured. He had had to make a pancake landing in the mountains, and he had escaped by scrambling out of his Piston Provost aircraft on to the wing, but not before he had been very badly burned, particularly on his hands. He had managed to crawl down the mountain in agony and had been found by a goatherd, who had got help from other locals. They had got him on a dhow to a local landing strip, but we were told he was in a bad way and wasn't likely to make it.

The Station Commander explained that the old landing strip in Muscat was set in a bowl in the hills, shaped for all the world like the crater of a volcano. It was a difficult landing for an aircraft at the best of times and had never been attempted at night. The only way of landing there was to fly through a narrow notch like a saddle on one side of the mountains and make a steep turning descent onto the sand runway. It took highly-skilled flying to land an aeroplane safely in that place at the best of times, and trying to land there in the dark on an unlit runway would be extremely dangerous. He was emphatic that he could not allow anyone to fly in there at night.

However, one team pilot and navigator from 152 Squadron, anxious to do all they could to rescue a fellow pilot, insisted that they were willing to try it. In the end the boss relented, on condition that any attempt at landing was delayed until the first light of dawn was beginning to show. I knew from the reports coming in from Muscat that the pilot was in a very bad state and feared that even the slightest delay in getting him out would jeopardise his chances of survival. I volunteered to join the flight and use my medical skills to accompany the injured pilot back to Bahrain. Ian Mercer was very unhappy with this proposal, but he reluctantly agreed to let me accompany them, emphasising that it was against his better judgement.

We set off in pitch darkness, hoping and praying that there would be enough light to enable us to land. By the time we got close to our destination, the sun was not yet up and try as we might, we couldn't make out the saddle in the mountain, far less the little landing strip. I was getting a little anxious about the effect of a delay on my injured patient.

Then, almost like a miracle, light appeared on the horizon, just enough for us to identify the narrow opening in the mountain range and the outline of the airstrip beyond. Thanks to the unbelievable skills of the pilot and navigator, we managed to touch down safely and get our injured pilot aboard.

He was in a bad way and kept asking about his hands, because he was a very accomplished pianist and was worried that he would never be able to play again. Our concern was simply to keep the poor man alive long enough to get him home and give him some treatment. We thought we had lost him a couple of times on the flight back, but we got him into the Government Hospital in Bahrain and he survived.

Sadly that wonderful navigator was less fortunate; he was killed not long afterwards, when he clipped a wing in his twin Pioneer and somersaulted. All but one on board were killed instantly.

After that incident I had to deal with widespread rumours about the effects of repeated washing on the men's flying suits. The word had got round that the frequent washing required by hot desert conditions destroyed the fireproofing and left aircrew vulnerable to burns in the event of an accident. I knew that couldn't be true, as in reality there was no fireproofing as such, but the men believed that frequent washing would actually increase the risk of spreading flames. Despite the lack of evidence they would not be reassured.

There was only one way to find out the answer to this and allay anxiety in the aircrew. I carried out some experiments, comparing the effects of fire on the fabric from a new suit with one that had been washed many times. As far as I could see, there seemed to be no difference. I asked for a full suit to experiment on and at first this was refused, but the CO overruled the objections and arranged for me to have one new suit, plus one which had been washed very many times.

I summoned some of the crew to a demonstration on a patch of desert on the airfield periphery and had two life-size dummies made from plaster of Paris (they were nicknamed POP for obvious reasons) to 'model' the two suits. Then I set fire to them. When we lit them, there was no difference whatsoever between the two suits; they both burned at the same rate. It seemed to satisfy the members of the squadrons, and it was a clear reminder of the value of demonstrating one's findings. POP, who remained intact during the demonstration, was adopted by one of the squadrons as their mascot and was wheeled out from time to time to participate in some of their social evenings.

Not long after that incident I was asked to investigate an outbreak of boils occurring in pilots of the Sultan of Oman's air force in Muscat. The crews were blaming everything they could think of for the outbreak, including the water, the food and a host of other possibilities, none of which made sense to me. I took a flight down to their base in Bait al Falaj in Muscat to investigate the problem.

Using the technique I had developed for field trials and investigations I shadowed them for days, even joining them on operational flights into the desert. I observed that when the pilots got ready to go out to their aircraft they would grab at random one of several flying suits hanging in their crew changing room. Unlike most other squadron pilots, they did not have their own dedicated suit. I also noticed that on return from their operations they would stand under the shower wearing the sweaty flying suit, which was then left to dry out on one of the pegs. It was clear that the cold water shower was inadequate to kill off the staphylococcal bacteria responsible for the outbreak of boils. It would only take one person with even a single boil to spread it on to the next pilot to wear the suit.

The suggestion that each pilot should have his own coverall was accepted, but the instruction to wash the flying suit frequently in boiling water did not go down well at first. The rumour that boiling would destroy flame retardance was still ripe among the pilots, as it was the recent crash in which one of their crew members had been so badly burned which had spawned the rumours.

Eventually I persuaded them that there was no foundation for their fears and my advice was accepted. I was glad to hear later that they had no problems with boils thereafter. It was a very simple investigation, but a satisfying one nonetheless, and it showed that in applied medicine and field trials you don't need sophisticated equipment to obtain a good result.

My interest in cars continued while I was in the Middle East and about this time I bought my first American vehicle. I had been warned that one of my predecessors had bought a new Volvo, which he hoped to take home with him at the end of his tour of duty. He stripped off all the brightwork and meticulously covered each item with gauze and Vaseline, putting it all into dry storage so he could replace it on the car before taking it home. Despite all his efforts to preserve his new car, the climate of Bahrain took its toll and he was left with a collection of beautiful shiny chromium and a rusting shell of bodywork, brittle as a biscuit with rust and with no way of securing the chrome fittings back on the car. He had to leave it out there when he returned.

That showed me that it wasn't worth wasting a lot of money on a new car out in the Middle East. Instead I went looking for something more cheap and cheerful, and on a second-hand car site I found a splendid Plymouth Savoy V8 and bought it on the spot. I had great fun in that car - until two pilots from the Hunter Squadron asked to borrow it for a few days while their own vehicle was being repaired. I forgot to tell them that the Plymouth's radiator leaked like a sieve. They forgot to top up the water in the cooling system, and of course, the engine seized. A replacement engine was too expensive to consider, so it was a write-off. After that I had to use an RAF Land Rover, but at least I hadn't lost much money.

When it was time to take our annual leave entitlement we could either fly back to the UK or go to one of the leave centres in East Africa. The choice was either Nairobi or Mombasa. I had heard quite hair-raising tales of the goings-on there by the troops let loose in Mombasa, so I chose Nairobi. It was a wise choice I think, as I was able to see Amboseli Game Park, which was a wonderful experience.

I tried to book into the famous Treetops Hotel, where Princess Elizabeth was staying in February 1952 when she got news that her father King George the Sixth had died and she had become Queen. Needless to say, with that association the hotel was fully booked and had been for months, so I had to make do with a rather less exotic but nonetheless pleasant hotel just outside Nairobi. It consisted of individual thatched sleeping huts laid out in a circle with the dining and lounge areas placed in the centre - just like an African village compound. The huts were comfortable but basic and the bed was covered by a canopy of anti-mosquito netting. Despite this precaution I was glad that I had taken all the necessary antimalarial pills.

I had a nasty moment when I awoke during an afternoon siesta to find a huge spider walking slowly across the canopy above me. I had no idea whether it was poisonous or not and I was taking no chances, so I leapt out of bed, shot through the hut door and tumbled out on to the dusty ground of the compound. I never was very keen on creepy crawlies at the best of times, and after that incident the thought that poisonous spiders and possibly snakes could come into the hut kept me awake for hours.

My only other encounter with African wildlife was when I was on a guided tour of the game park. The guide took us on a walk along the river bank to see some hippopotami wallowing in the muddy river. At one point we had to cross a swampy area where the pathway split to give us two alternative crossings. The guide indicated the pathway we should take, but I stupidly chose to take my own route and tried to cross using some logs which looked like convenient stepping stones.

As I was about to put my foot down, I got the shock of my life. One of the logs moved slightly and I caught a glimpse of a large crocodile eye glowering angrily at me. For the second time on that holiday I had to make a jump to save my skin!

I was taking no chances, as these beasts were notorious for attacking and killing villagers who came down to the river for water. I don't think the old crocodile was particularly interested in having me for his lunch, and after the disturbance of his morning nap, he lazily went back to sleep.

It was absolute bliss to taste the food in Kenya. The fresh milk, bacon and eggs and bananas for breakfast were in stark contrast to the Bahrain diet of powdered milk and thinly-sliced beef (which took the place of bacon) served up with reconstituted powdered eggs. There were, of course, no deep freezers at that time and the supplies which came in on the weekly VC10 aircraft were very limited indeed.

While I was there I took the opportunity to visit RAF Eastleigh, just outside Nairobi. The Senior Medical Officer there had a Land Rover staff car like mine and very kindly showed me round the local area. Unfortunately just as we approached the main gate to the airfield on our return, the engine packed up and we had to walk several hundred yards to the guardhouse to get some assistance. By the time we got back with a retrieval party some 20 minutes later, the Land Rover had been stripped completely; all the seats, tyres and everything else which might be useful to the locals had been pinched. There was almost nothing left but a sorry-looking shell of a vehicle. I was sorry for my medical colleague who would have to explain the loss of Service property, but he told me this kind of thing was forever happening and he wasn't too worried.

When I returned to Bahrain after my leave, my third and final experiment was with parachutists who were coming in for treatment for some nasty landing injuries. I asked the parachute medical officer what he thought could be going wrong, but he could not explain it. These men were highly trained, yet they were repeatedly suffering leg, ankle and back injuries from routine jumps.

I flew out with them in a Beverley and watched them jumping and landing in the drop zone. I actually tried to get permission to jump with them, but I was refused, and told I would be in serious trouble if I tried it. The Parachute

Regiment came up with a good solution. They would teach me basic landing techniques using two mess tables piled one on top of the other. When I managed to master the very basic techniques of landing they taught me to use a special parascending parachute used by the Regiment as a training tool as well as for recreation purposes.

Once I got to grips with the technique I became quite adept at donning the harness and running as fast as my legs would carry me at the end of a towrope attached to the back of an accelerating Land Rover. In the right conditions the round parachute would take me up to a good altitude, and when the winchman on the Land Rover signalled for me to disengage from the towline I would descend freely to the ground under the canopy. I tried this many times on one of the rarely-used runways and having learned the technique, I made a fairly decent show of landing on most occasions.

On one flight, however, I made a very poor landing and hurt my ankle. Unpleasant as that was, it gave me an idea as to the possible cause of the injuries we were seeing during practice drops in the desert. On that particular descent I had had a bad night's sleep and was quite switched off and not really feeling enthusiastic about the prospect of parascending but felt obliged to do so. It suddenly dawned on me that perhaps it was straightforward fatigue that was at the root of the problem.

I decided to look further into the matter. My experience in experimental analysis had taught me always to look for anything different from usual procedure, something test pilots did when a test flight did not go according to plan.

What was different here was that one of the two parachute units had the early morning take-off. Having prepared the night before and checked their equipment, they were given a few hours' rest time before taking off in the cool part of the day. However most of them didn't feel it worth going to bed for such a short time and played cards or chatted until it was time to be bussed out to the airfield to board the Beverley, so they had had no sleep.

That was it - these men were half asleep. They were switched off. When you are dozy and there is little adrenalin in your bloodstream, you don't perform any kind of task well, certainly not parachute jumping.

To prove my hunch, I designed a memory test based on one we had used at Farnborough. It required them to carry out a simple calculation, and when I tested them aboard the aircraft just before they reached the drop zone they performed badly when compared with a control group jumping at a different time of day. I asked two parachuting instructors to assess the quality of the landings in the DZ and like the memory test there was a marked difference between the early morning group and the others jumping later in the day.

Naturally, given the military culture, it would have been a hell of a job trying to persuade the army to change its routine and set aside a decent length of time for a night's sleep, but I gave the results of my findings to the RAMC Medical Officer who looked after 2 and 3 Parachute Regiment. Somehow he managed to do some persuading, and I had the satisfaction of noting that from then on the injury rate reduced to expected levels.

One job we had to do was take over from Medical Officers at other Middle Eastern bases as locums while they were on leave, which gave me a chance to see something of Muscat and Dubai. I was able to spend three weeks in Muscat, where the Sultan of Oman's Air Force (SOAF) was based, on the old airfield there. At that time, it was used to support his army and was mainly locally staffed with RAF aircrew on detachment.

I had the chance to do pretty much all the flying I wanted, and I was in my element. We used Piston Provosts and Canadian de Havilland Beavers as spotter planes, with RAF pilots on detachment, and they let me fly these aircraft. They had a trainer Provost, and I got my hands on it on every possible occasion.

We had a problem at that time with unscrupulous Arabs in dhows who were picking up pilgrims to Mecca, taking their money and then dumping them on the sand and telling them Mecca was 'just over there' when in fact it was well over a thousand miles away to the west. Many of these poor people perished in the desert. We had to pinpoint where these crooks' dhows were landing and fly up the camel routes to look for people in distress, then alert the Army to pick them up. We were doing this one day when we heard the faint but unmistakeable 'whoosh' of rifle bullets zipping past the aircraft. We were being shot at from one of the old Portuguese forts that were dotted about the area. It was a worrying moment, but those missions gave me a tremendous insight into operational flying and brought me some real flying experience.

My next locum detachment was to the airfield and base at Sharjah, which had started life as a primitive landing strip and refuelling point used by the old Imperial Airways for intercontinental stopovers. During World War 2 the base had been extended and it had eventually come under the administration of RAF Bahrain.

On arrival there, it became clear that I would be brushing up on my medical casualty work; there were many head-on collisions along the straight, fast road between Sharjah and nearby Dubai. The living accommodation there was rather crude and we had to use salt-water showers, which were almost worse than not having a shower at all as you came out feeling stickier than you were when you went in. Even the use of salt-water soap helped very little.

My flying skills were put to the test one day when a camel walked right across the runway just as I was about to land. I was using the opportunity of a quiet airfield and empty airspace to catch up on the air experience training which at that time every Doctor in the RAF was expected to undergo. Under the supervision of a very experienced pilot-in-command I was about to make my first attempt at landing a Twin Pioneer aircraft. As a comparative learner I had little experience of dealing with such an emergency and I only just managed to complete the landing safely without hitting the poor animal. The Captain was much relieved, if a little shaken, but the incident served to convince him that Medical Officers and flying do not make a good combination. It taught me, however, to be more vigilant in future.

I was holding a medical clinic in the Sharjah centre one morning when a group of Arabs charged in and asked me to come outside. They were escorting no less a personage than the ruling Sheik, who was watching proceedings from his hunting vehicle, an open-topped long-wheelbase Land Rover. His chief falconer had brought an injured hunting hawk with him. He showed it to me; it had a deep gash on one of its feet. 'You mend!' he said. It sounded more like an order than a request, and I lost no time in inspecting the casualty.

I felt somewhat put on the spot, as I had no knowledge of bird husbandry. I scratched my head for a moment and then decided to apply some Aureomycin cream, a very powerful antibiotic. I smeared some of the bright yellow cream on the bird's foot, gave the falconer the tube and suggested that he should apply repeat doses for the next few days. I was a little nervous, as I had visions of getting my hand chopped off if the hawk died. However the falconer seemed satisfied with my treatment of the bird and after deep conversation with the Sheik watching from his car indicated that I could take a photograph of the two of us with his favourite hawk. Sad to say, I had no camera on me at the time and the opportunity to get a snapshot of the incident was lost.

After much bowing and waving the hunting party left, and I can only presume that my treatment was spot on and the bird recovered.

However, this was not quite the end of the story. Hearing of my encounter with the Sheik and the bird, Flying Officer 'Puddy' Catt, the Station Administration Officer, filed a joke report that a 'Jeff Hawk' had been seen by the Station Medical Officer and had been pronounced unfit to fly, having injured his leg. We all laughed at the joke, but some idiot managed to file it as a flying incident report and it trickled its way through to HQ Middle East Command in Aden. They wanted to know who this injured pilot was, but eventually accepted the explanation that the message they received must have been corrupted in transmission and that in any case it referred only to a 'paper exercise' in casualty evacuation we had carried out recently. No more about the incident was heard after that.

Back in Bahrain, the routine work continued. I was beginning to miss the real research work at Farnborough and wondering if I would ever make it to IAM. Then one day we had an inspection by the AOC (Air Officer Commanding) and I laid out a demonstration of the work I had been doing.

'Why are you not at Farnborough?' he asked me. A good question. But this proved to be an opportune encounter, because the AOC said he would have a word with someone, and the result was that my time in the Middle East came to an early and not unwelcome end. I was told I was being posted to the Aeromedical Training Centre at RAF Upwood in Cambridgeshire. This would be right up my street, because it involved training aircrew in the flying protective assemblies I had been working on at IAM.

As a preliminary to leaving and before handing over my inventory for the Emergency Medical Unit to the doctor who would be replacing me, the Wing Commander Senior Medical Officer asked me to take a team out to the far side of the airfield and set up the tented unit. The main object of the exercise was to see what we had left over from the Kuwait crisis. We put up marquees, set up kitchens and even erected an emergency treatment tent. We opened crate after crate of instruments which were rusted beyond use and fit only for the dustbin. There was no sign of the two Land Rover ambulances listed on the inventory, and they joined the growing list of items we got official permission to write off.

One item we didn't include in that list was a packing case full, of all things, of tins of rich fruit cake. Our airman cook had plans to use them, and after checking with me that the contents were still edible he set to the creation of a culinary masterpiece. He marinated the slices of cake in Drambuie which he had got hold of in the NAAFI, using the pretext that it would kill off any lingering bacteria (there were none of course). It was delicious, but extremely high octane, and we named his new recipe 'BAPCO pudding' after the local oil refinery in the area. The sight of tipsy men doing eightsome reels in the desert sand must have puzzled the Arabs who from the start of our exercise had been watching our every move through binoculars from the road outside the camp.

A few nights before my departure, the members of the Officers' Mess laid on a farewell party for me. It promised to be quite a lively event, complete with a guitar band and splendid buffet. The squadron had flown in enough red wine to float a battleship. They reputedly filled a spare fuel tank in one of their aircraft with it. Unfortunately it was 'coccinelle', which was dreadful stuff. It tasted quite bland and not too unpleasant to drink – until, that is, the after-effects set in. It was like being struck with a sledgehammer, and the dizziness was like a spiral dive in an aircraft. It made a ride in the disorientation trainer at IAM Farnborough like a walk in the park. The hangover effect of a night on the wine was quite unbelievable, and most people who had overindulged the night before temporarily lost the will to live.

Most of the bash took place outside in the Mess garden among the bougainvillea trees. But just as the party was getting into full swing, suddenly and without warning, the biggest rainstorm imaginable struck. Within moments everything was soaked. Cocktail treats lovingly prepared by the cooks and served by white-jacketed stewards turned into an unrecognisable mush. Peanuts floated from their dishes and water cascaded off the leaves of the bougainvilleas, diluting the abandoned glasses of wine. Of course the power went off, so that was the end of the garden lighting, and the electric guitars of the band died with a pathetic wail. People ran for cover into the shelter of the Mess building.

The rest of the party went off in the dark, which was inconvenient to say the least, except to some of the young female schoolteachers, who were getting on extremely well with the young flying officers. It was certainly turning out to be an evening I would never forget.

In fact it was one the world would never forget. It was November 22nd 1963 and in Dallas, Texas, a world-shattering event had just taken place. Just as the power had been restored at my farewell party and the celebrations had resumed, a signals officer came in to tell us that they had received a somewhat garbled message which seemed to indicate that the US President, John Kennedy, had been assassinated. There had been an immediate clampdown on communications, so we couldn't get any further news. Was the President really dead, or merely injured? Was it all a rumour? We had no way of knowing.

As it happened I had bought a cheap radio, because I wanted to put some Arab music on a tape to take back home with me. It didn't have much of a range, but inventive as usual, I rigged up an aerial with two coat hangers and started surfing the airwaves. I managed to pick up an American Forces Network broadcast from the US Air Force Base in Qatar, which confirmed the terrible news – the US President had been shot by an assassin on a visit to Dallas and had died of his injuries.

As I seemed to be the only one getting information, it fell to me to announce this news. I took notes from the radio bulletins and made several dashes over to the studio of Radio

RAF Bahrain, situated behind the Medical Centre. Putting on my best Richard Dimbleby voice, I was able to broadcast the tragic announcement to the rest of the station - my first real news broadcast. Shortly after that I was on a plane back home for Christmas.

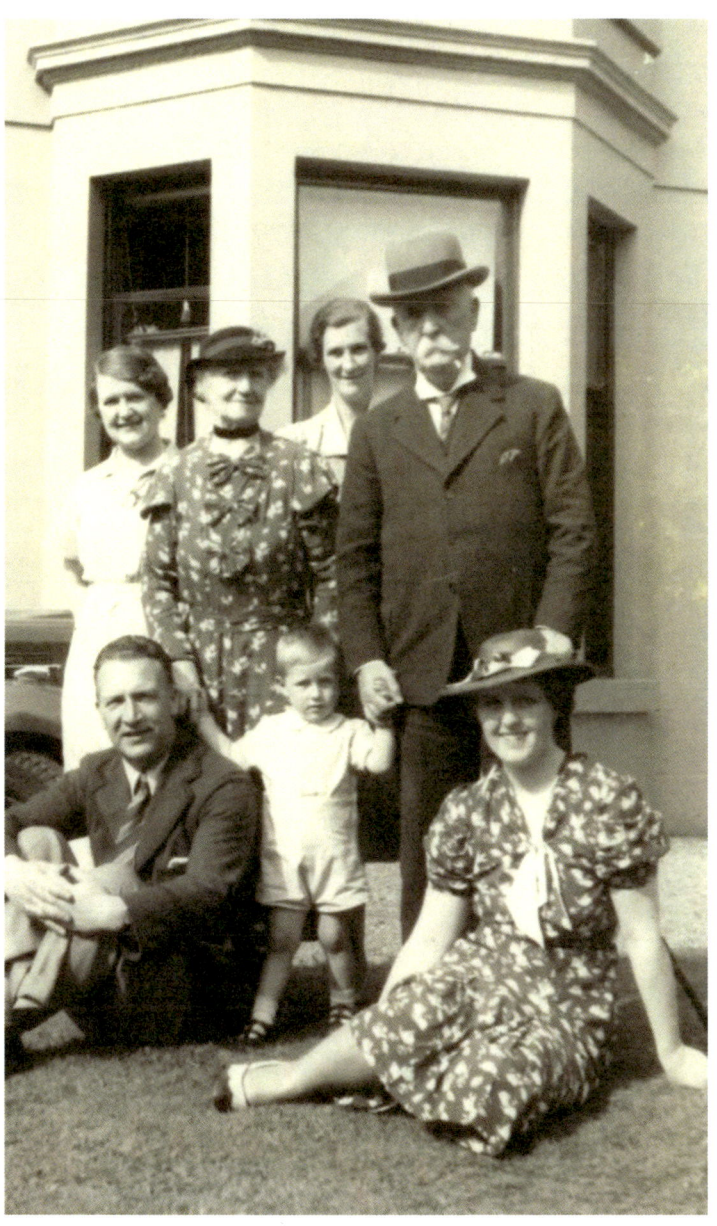

With my family outside Monkland, the family house which was destroyed in the Blitz. Standing: Auntie Nan, Granny Sharp, mother Mabel, Grandpa Sharp; seated are my father Russell, myself and cousin Joyce.

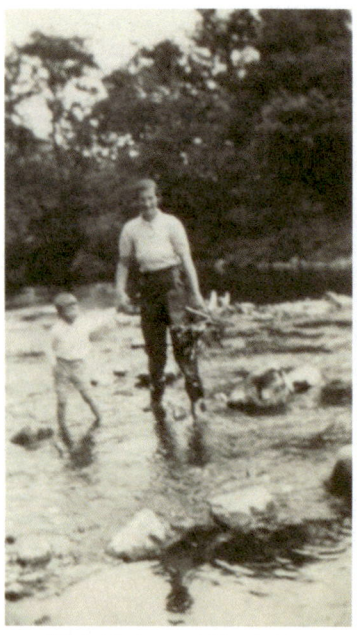

With Mother paddling in the River Earn below our holiday cottage in St Fillans.

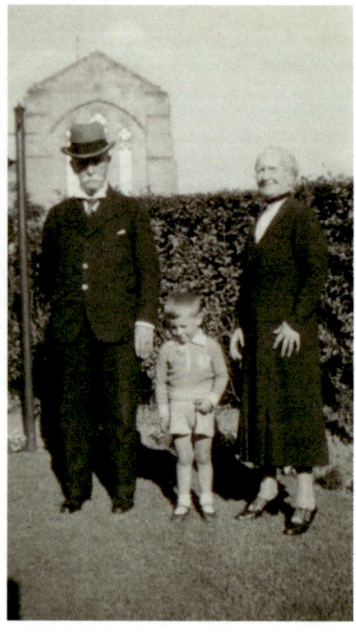

With Grandpa and Granny Sharp

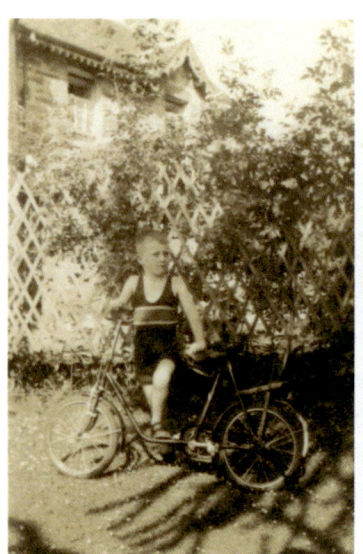

On two wheels…

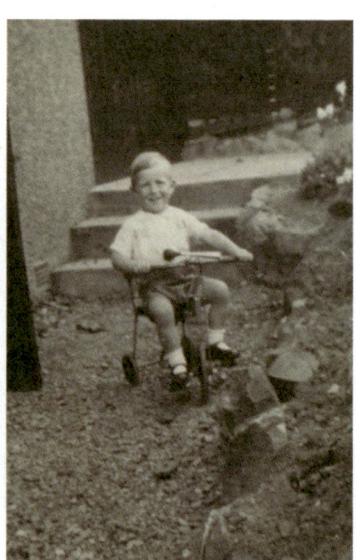

…and three…

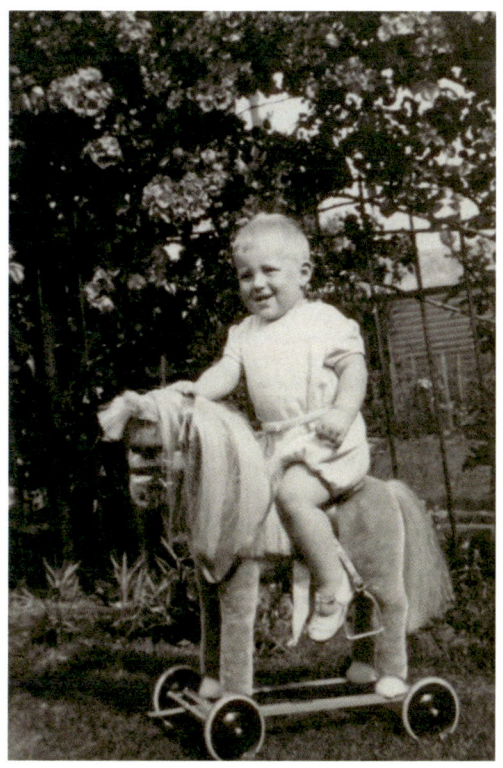
...and finally to four

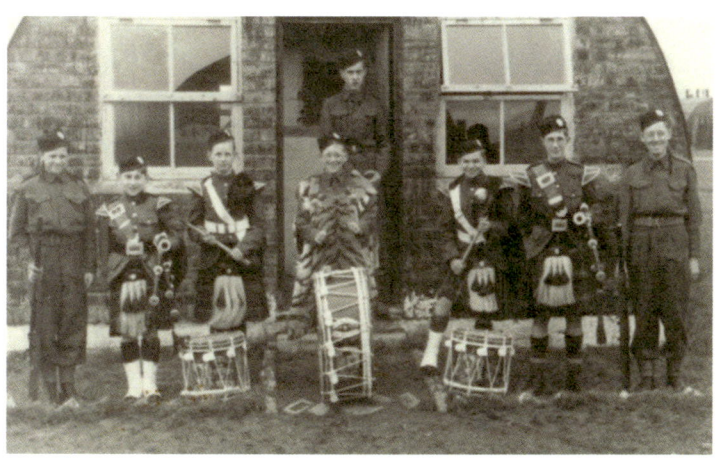
At annual CCF Camp, outside a Nissen hut.

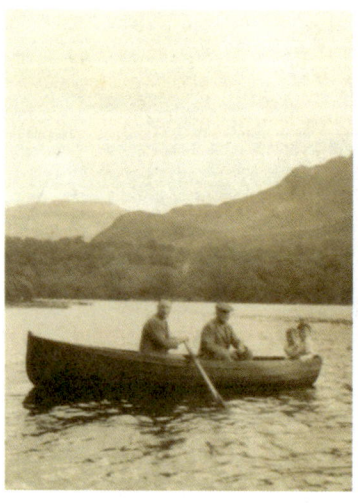

With my father, an uncle and a cousin fishing on Loch Earn.

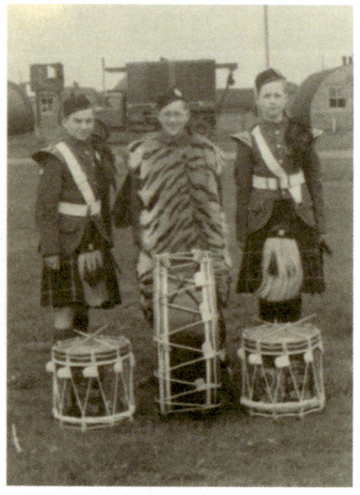

Playing the big drum in the Glasgow Academy Senior School Pipe Band with 'Mousy' Alexander (left) and 'Rosy' Reid (right).

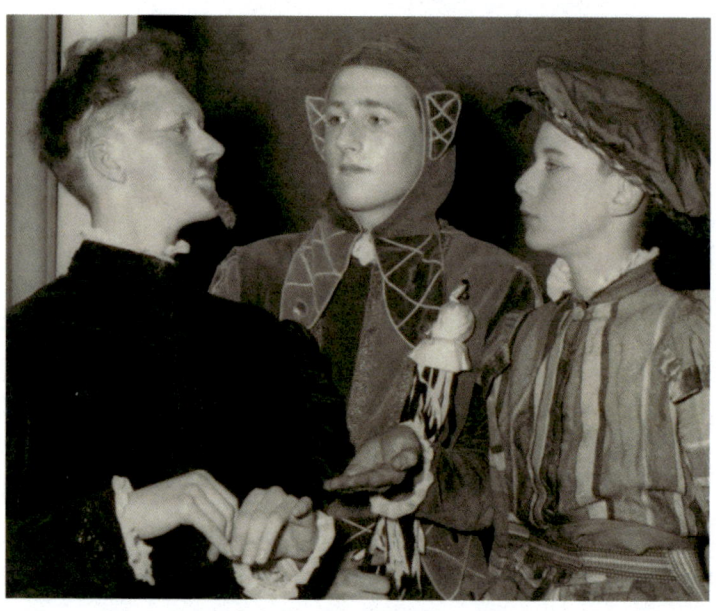

Playing Feste the Jester in a production of Twelfth Night by Glasgow Academy's Globe Players.

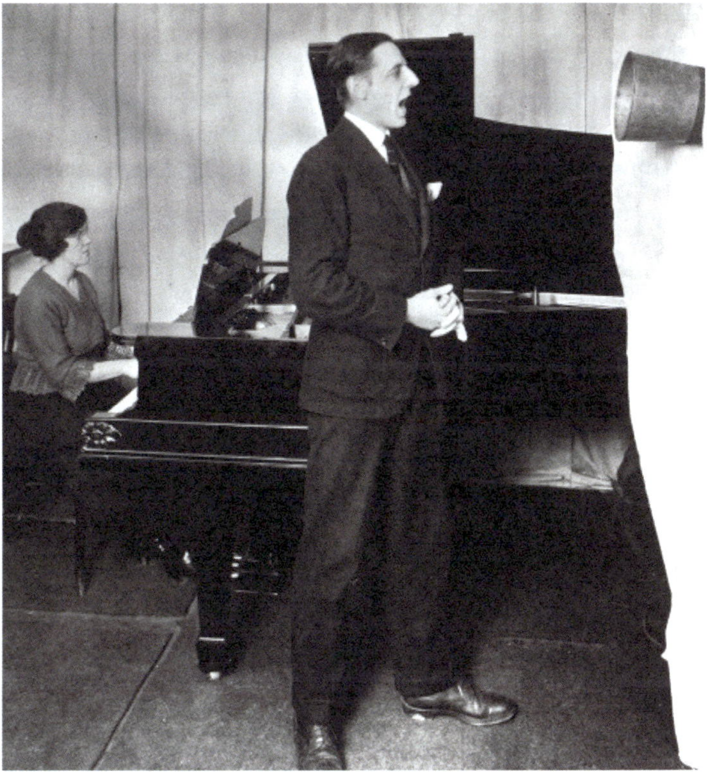

A performer at the BBC Manchester studios at Metrovick, where Dad worked.

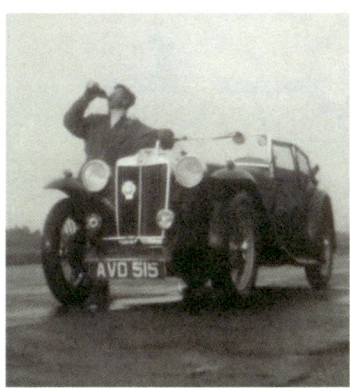

My dear friend Arthur Ferns with his MG TB at the old Balado Airfield (this is the car I ran into at University).

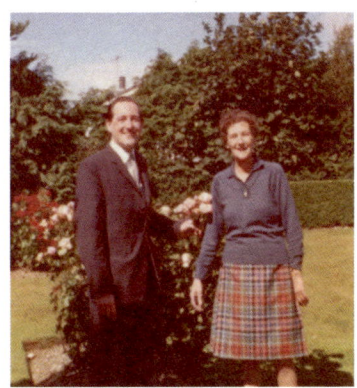

In Fortrose with Mother just after I had left Medical School.

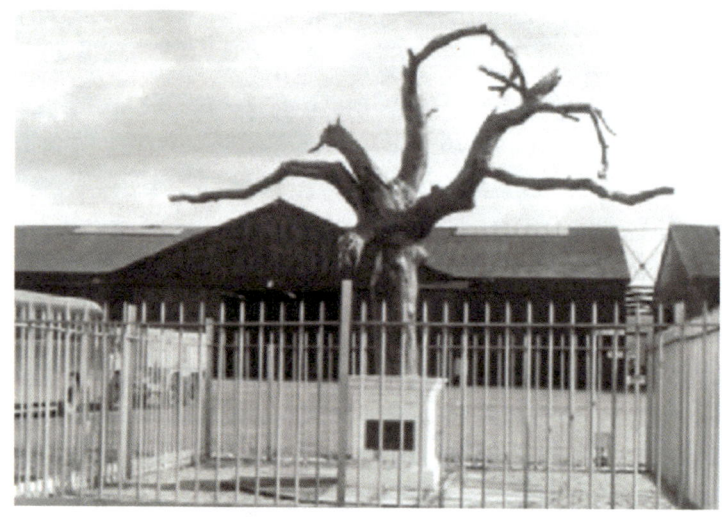
Cody's famous tree at Farnborough

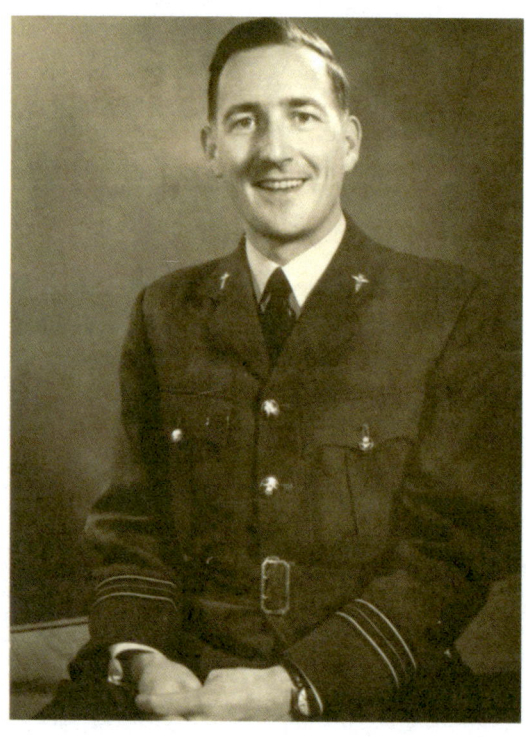
The author as a young RAF officer, early 1960s.

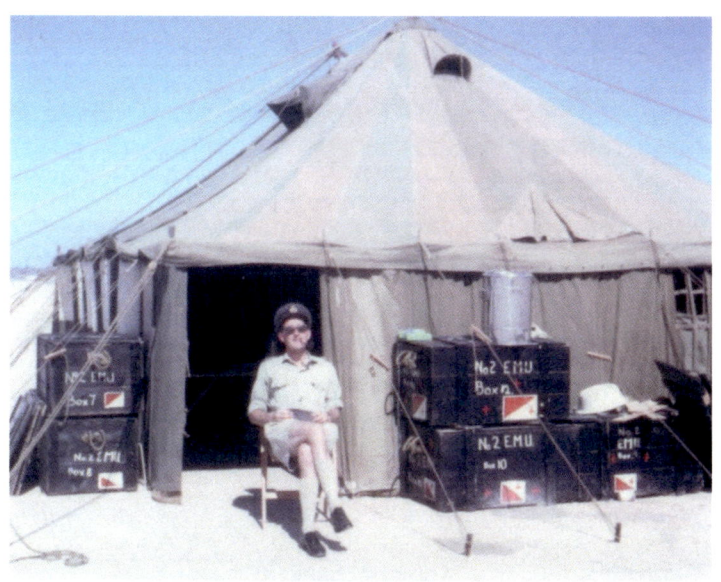

Setting up the EMU (Emergency Medical Unit) at Bahrain – it was last used in the Kuwait crisis.

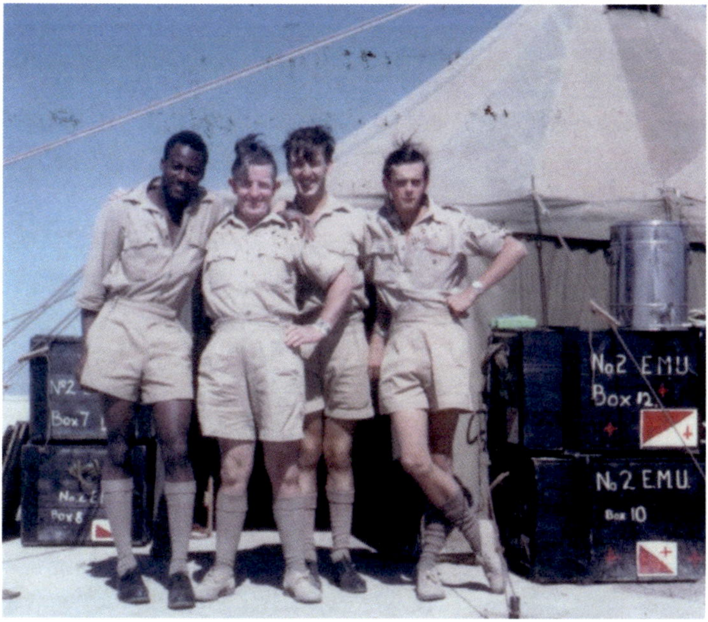

Members of the EMU team

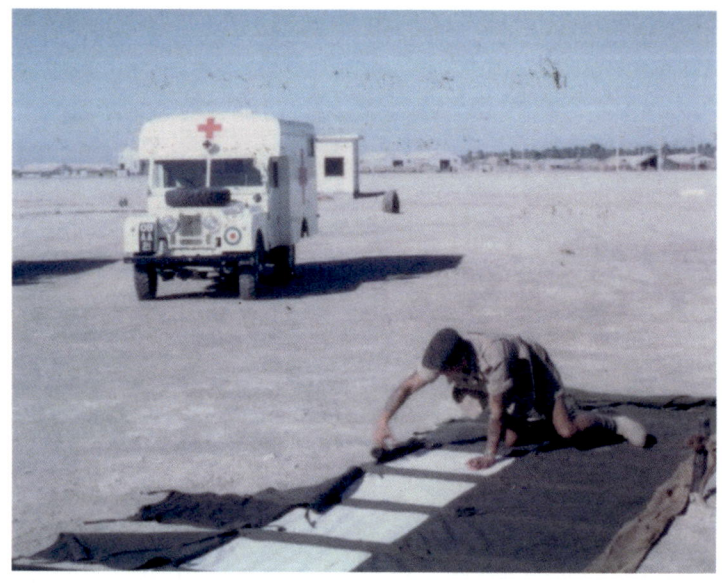

Setting up tents and marquees at EMU Bahrain

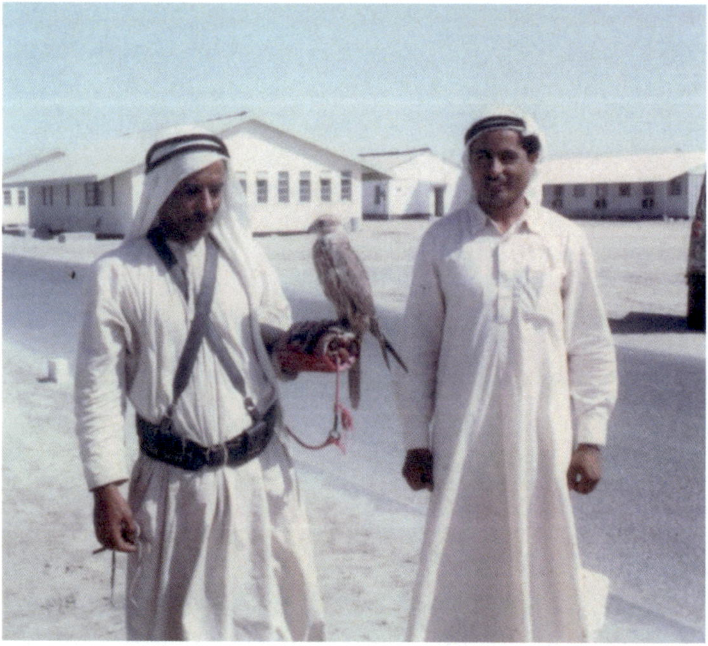

The hunting hawk brought in for treatment when I was at RAF Sharja

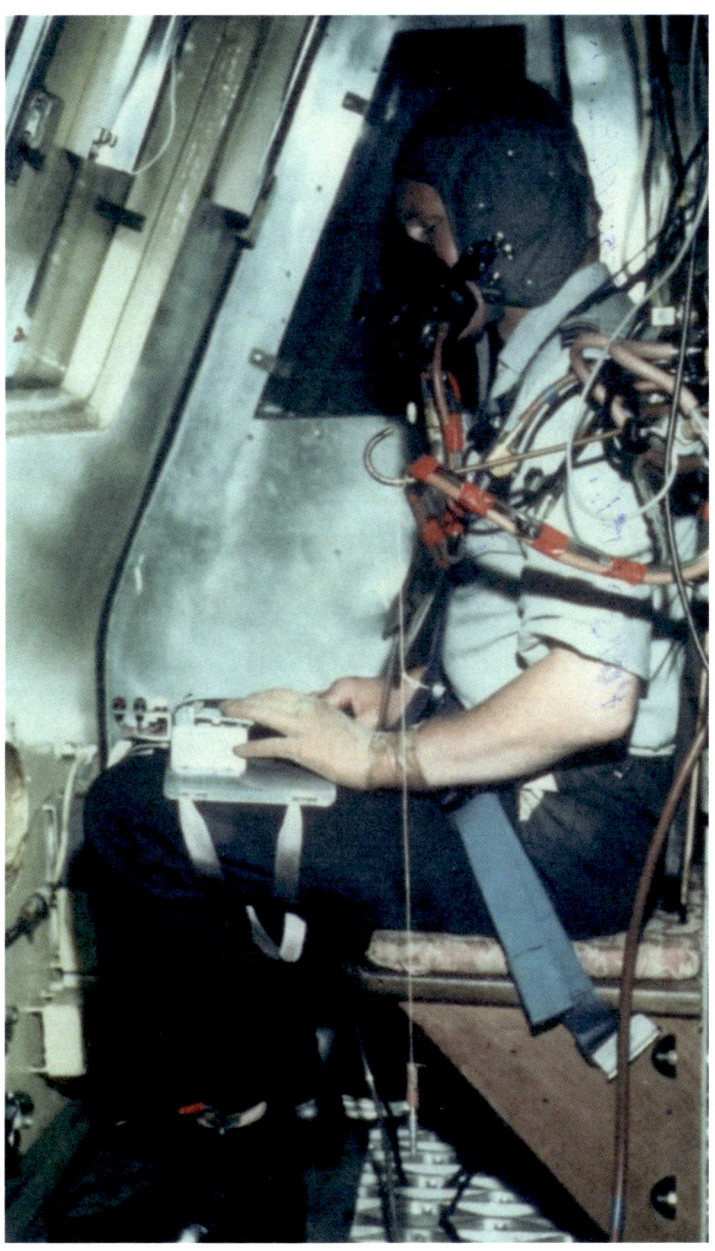

Don Cameron about to undergo rapid decompression in the high-performance chamber capsule.

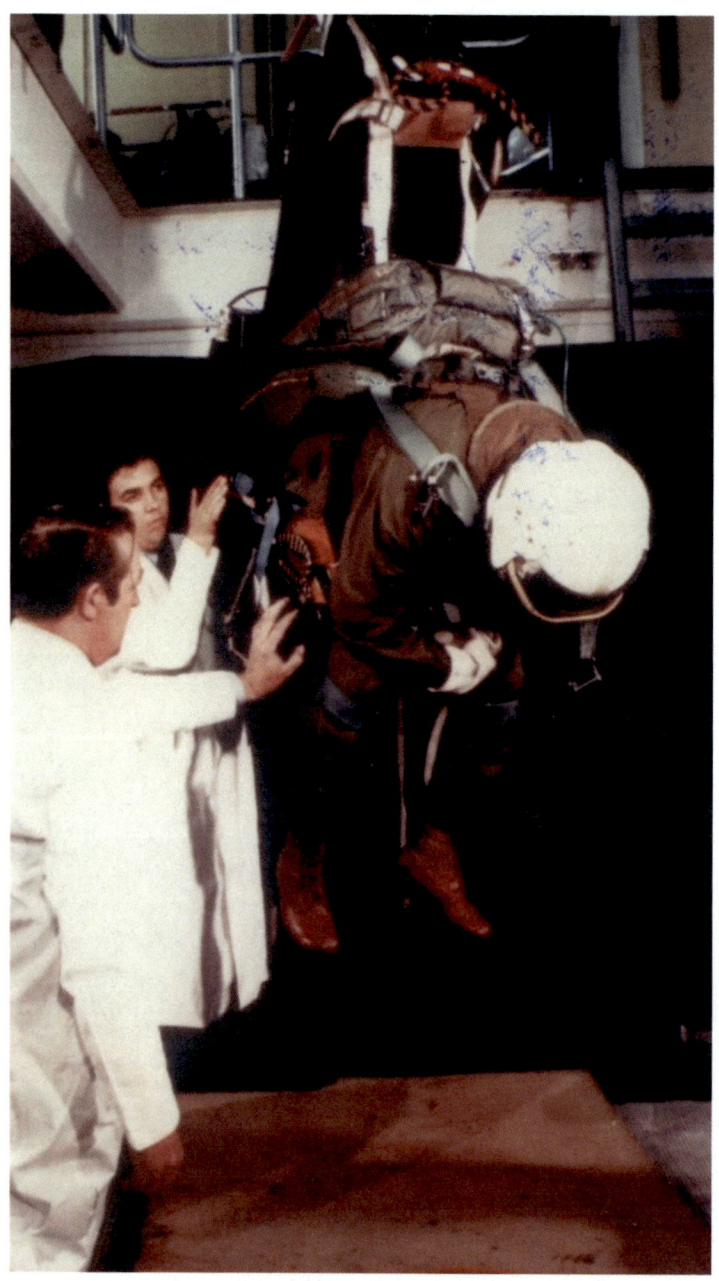

Testing a parachute harness

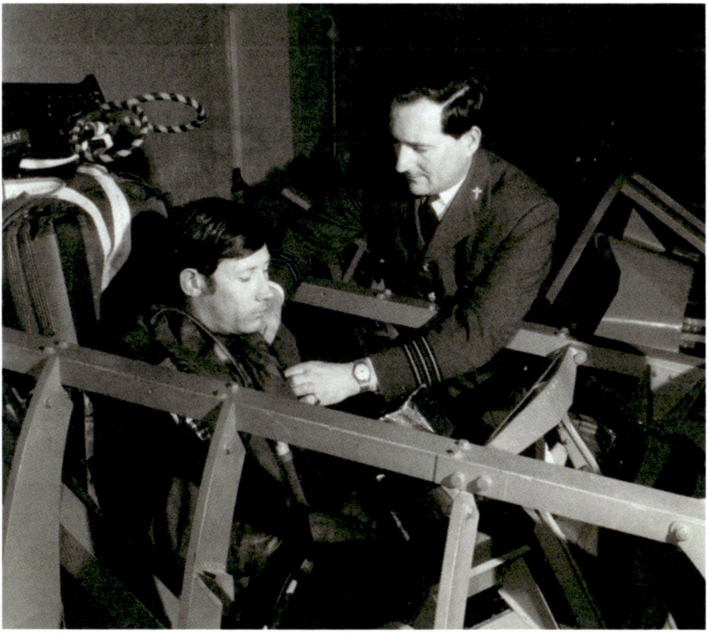

Assessing assemblies in a cockpit mock-up

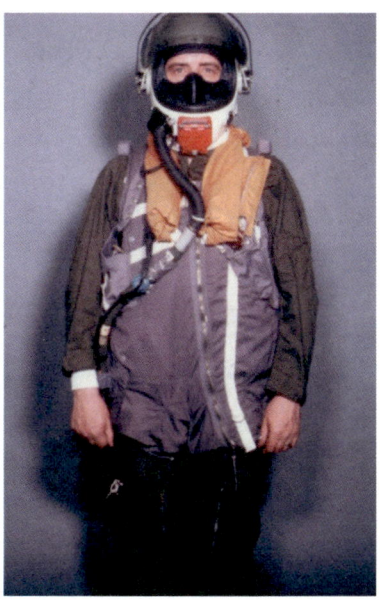

Protective assembly testing

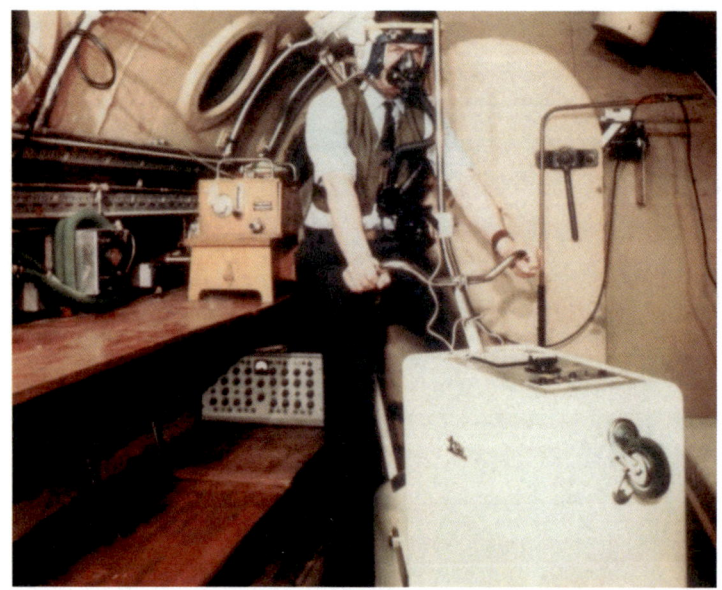

Protective assembly testing

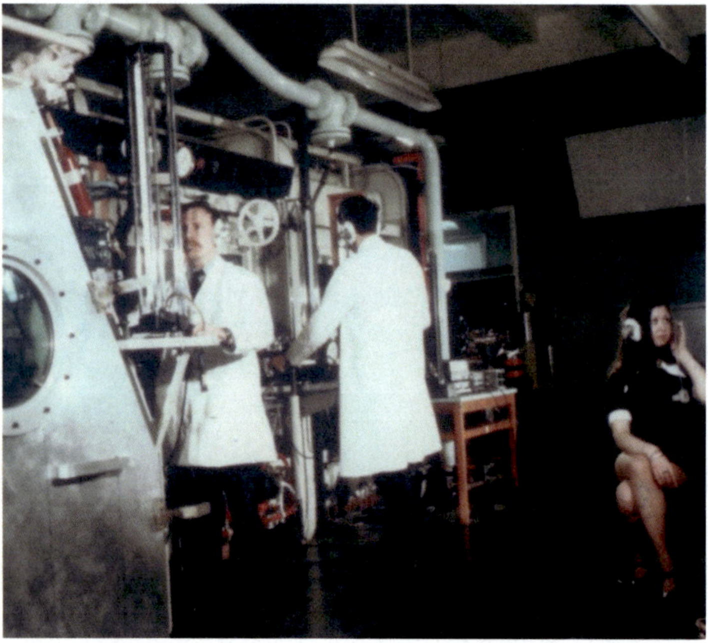

High performance decompression chamber, Altitude Division, IAM

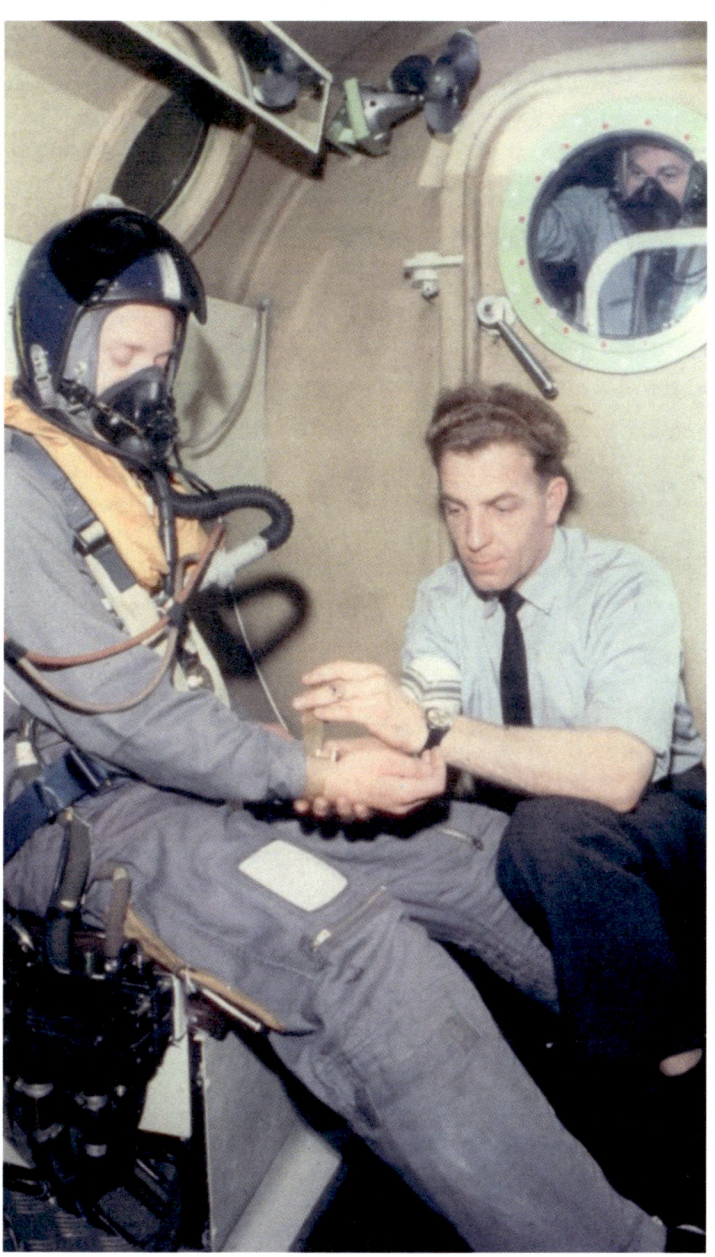

Preparing to conduct a hypoxia demonstration
(That's me at the window!)

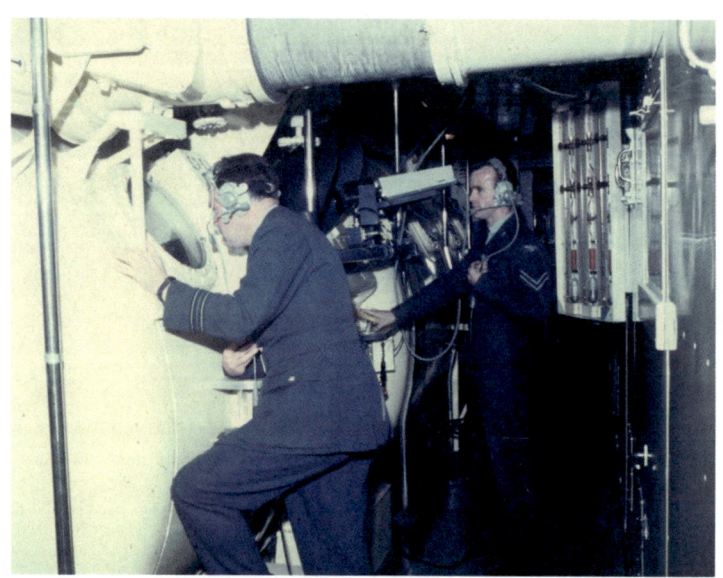

Testing the effects of loss of cabin pressure

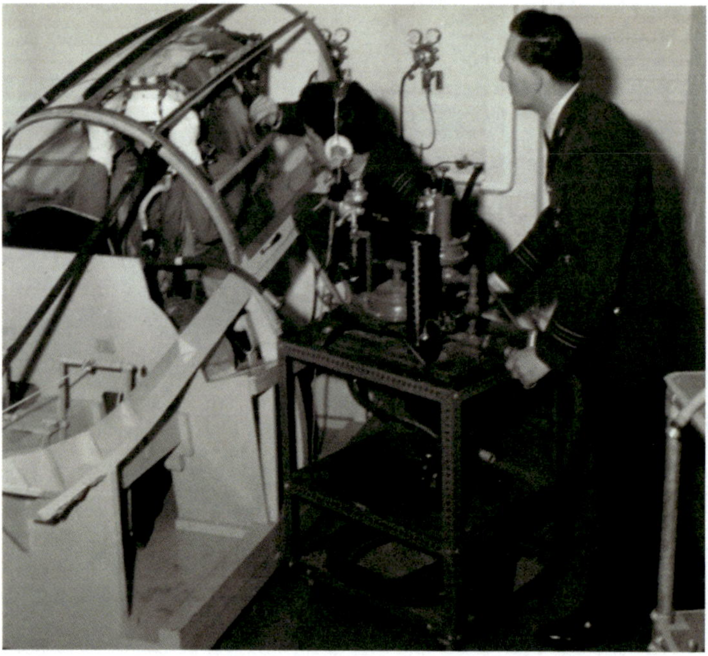

Testing protective assemblies in a cockpit mock-up

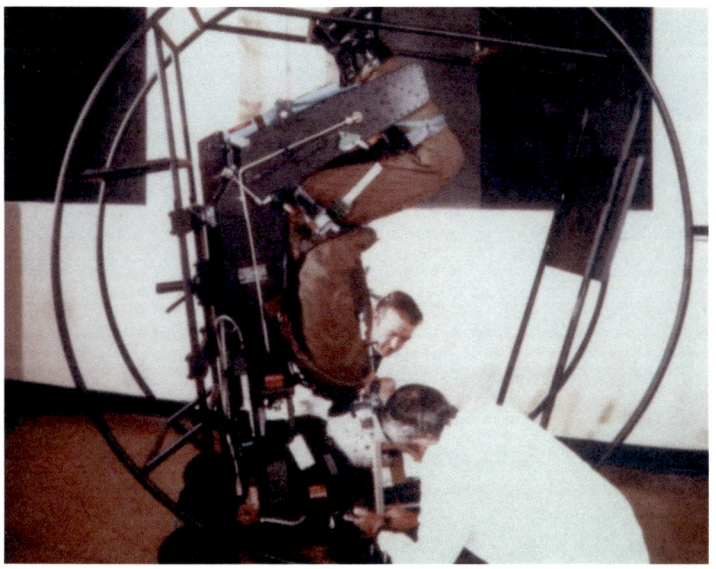

Oxygen equipment and protective assembly testing for escape in inverted flight

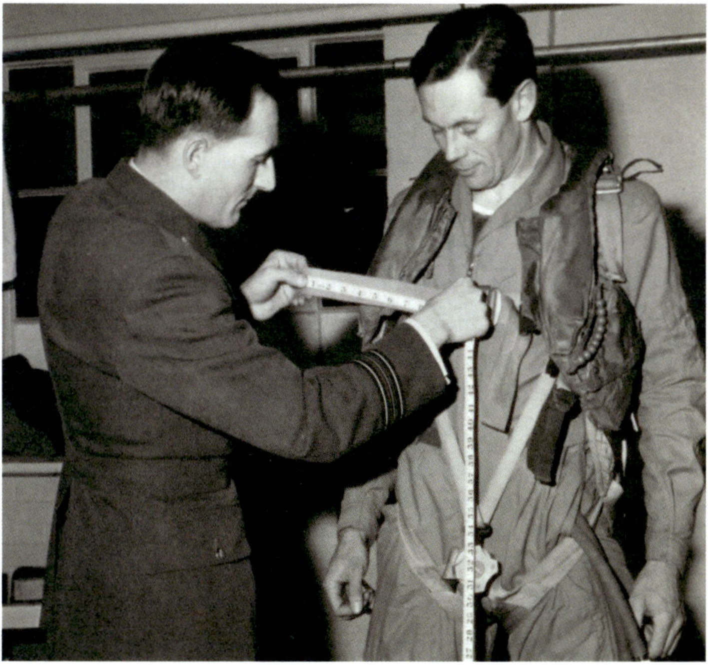

Fitting a parachute harness

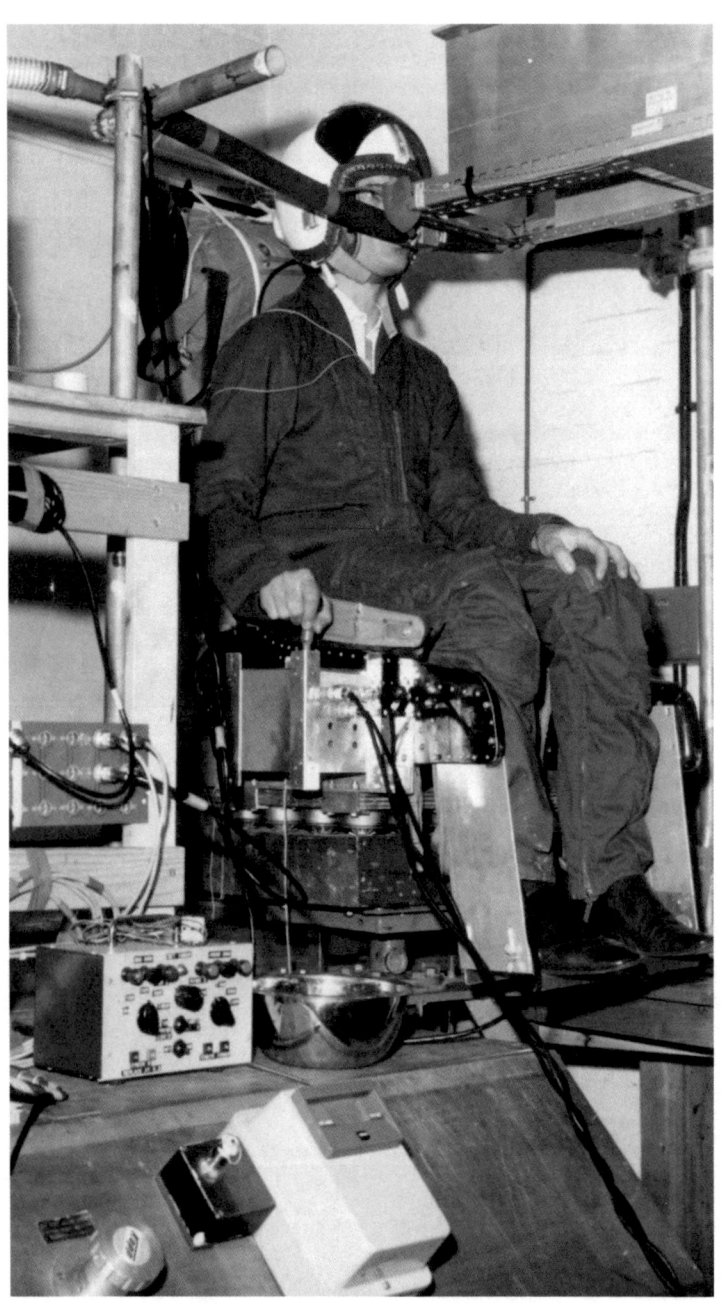

Experiment using the whole-body vibrator

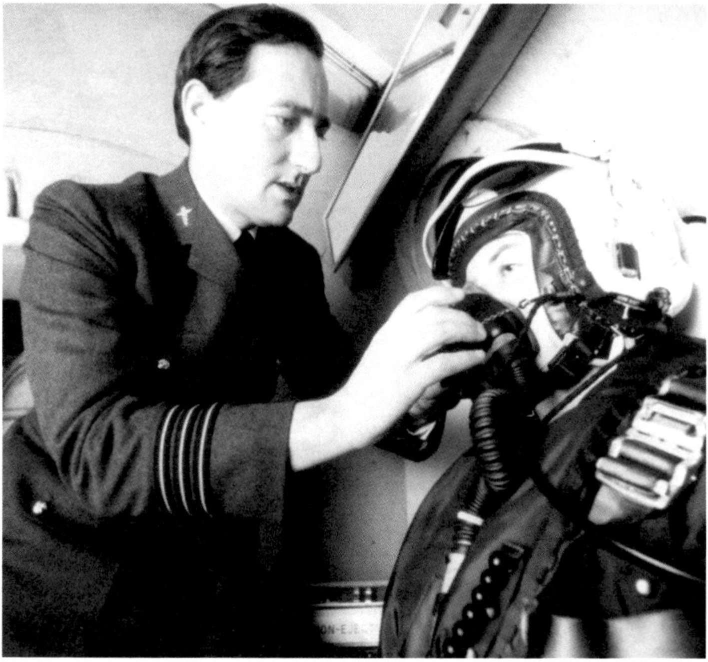

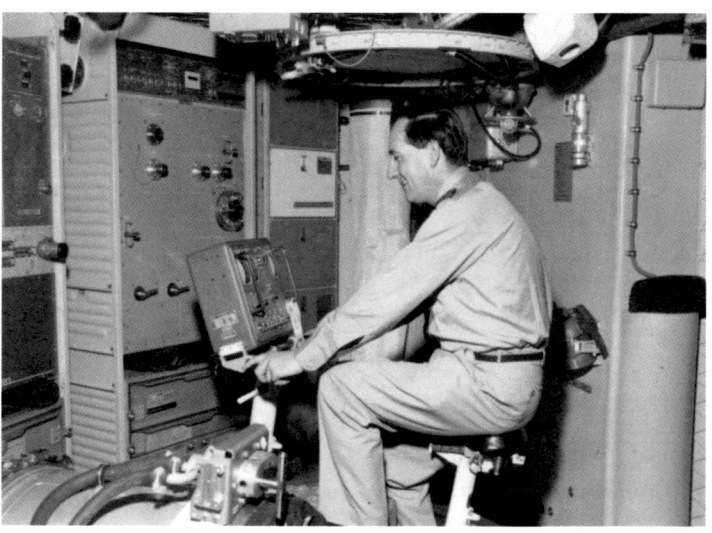

Demonstrating effects of hypoxia at simulated altitude in decompression chamber

Trying out an experiment in Skylab
(at the Manned Spacecraft Centre in Houston)

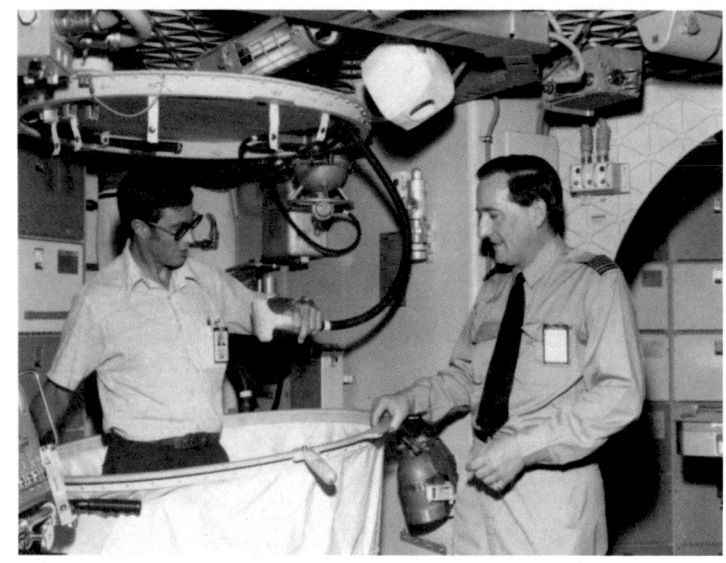

Mike Whittle demonstrates the shower on Skylab

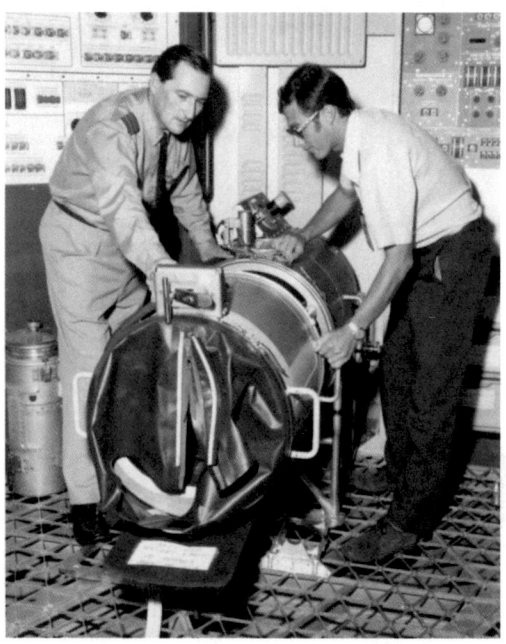

Examining the 'body box' used to assess Skylab astronauts' heart and circulation in space

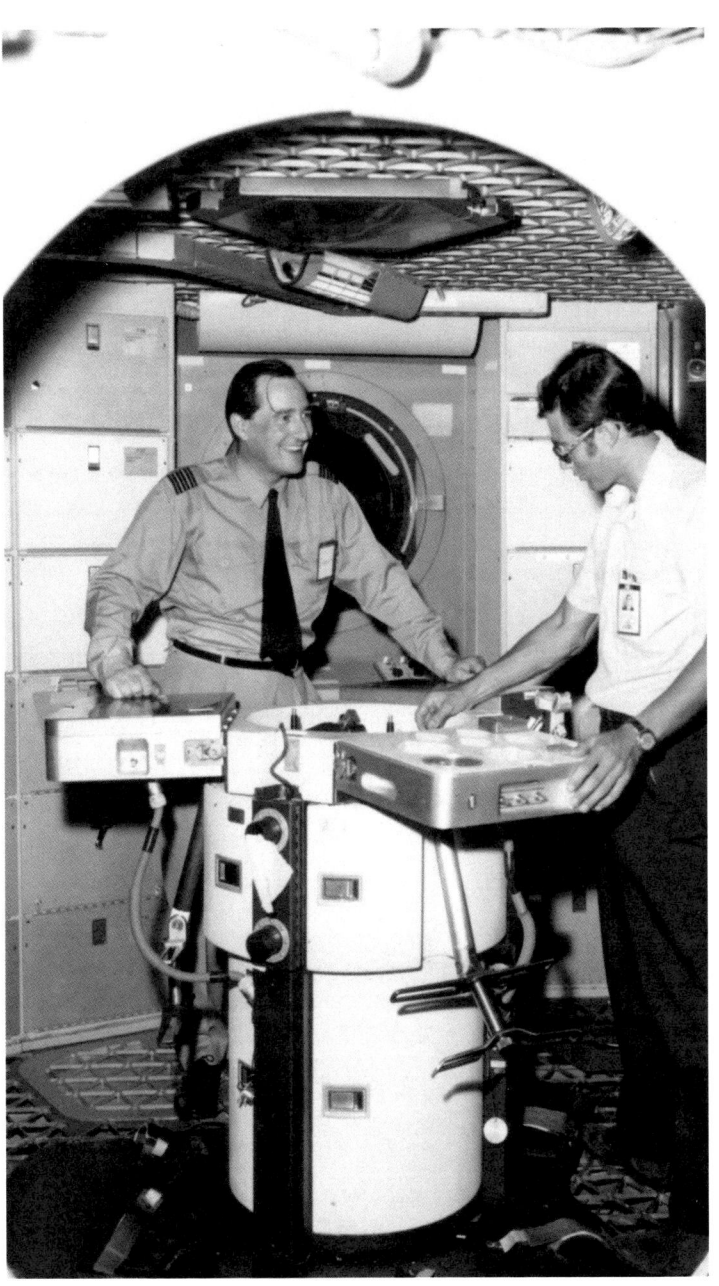

Skylab food preparation bay

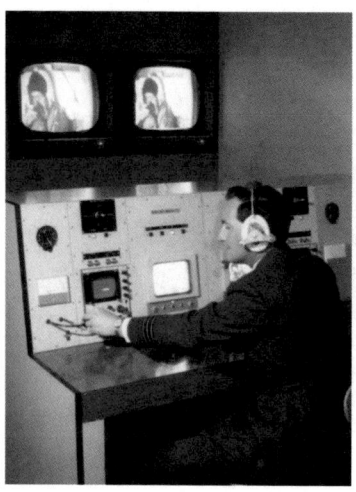

My mini 'Mission Control' at AMTC – monitoring aircrew during rapid decompression (it was based on my visit to NASA Mission Control).

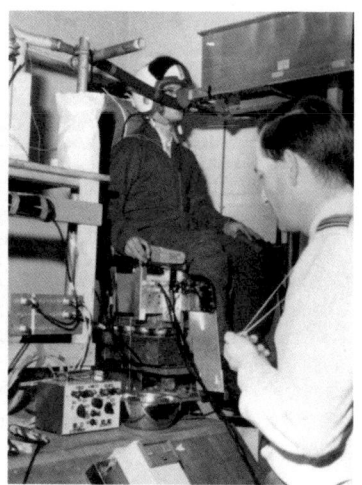

Whole body vibration experiments at IAM

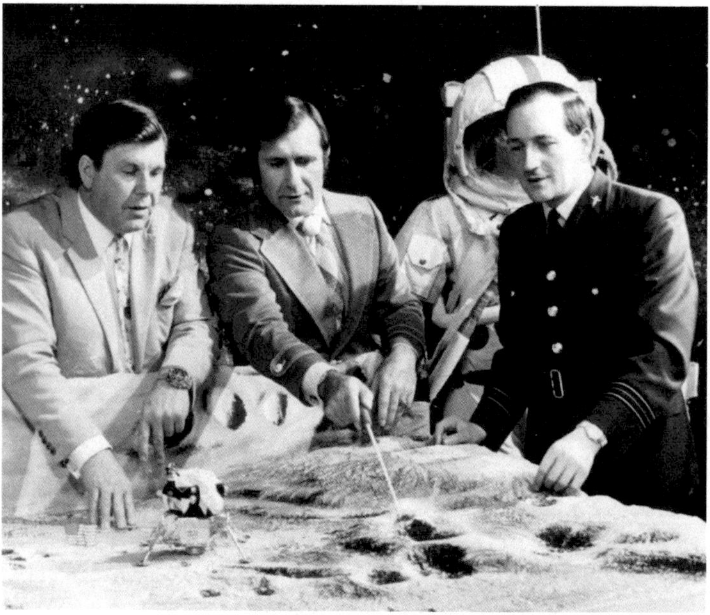

An Apollo 14 broadcast at ITN with Peter Fairley (left) and astronaut Dick 'cowboy' Gordon.

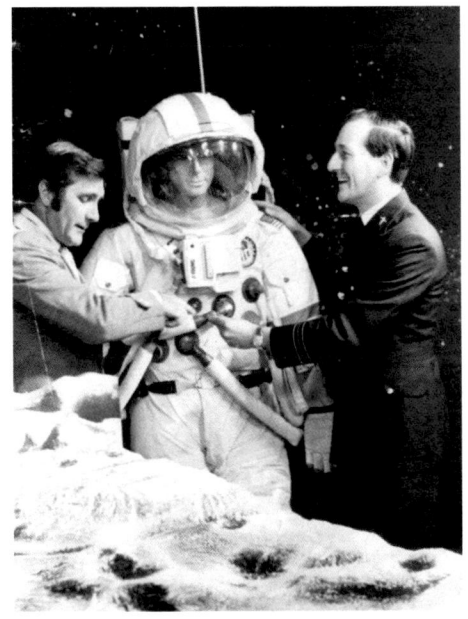

Dick Gordon helps me to explain to viewers how the astronauts' pressure suits work.

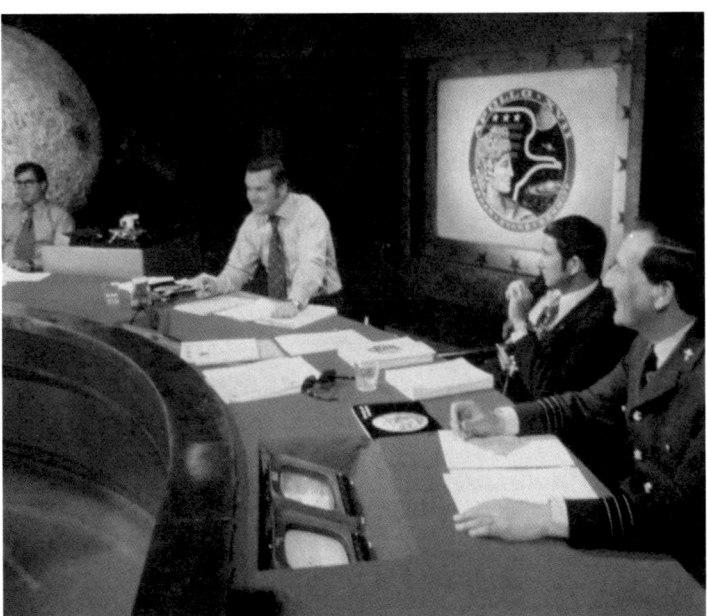

In the studio of ITN during the Apollo 17 mission. Left to right: Peter Fairley, Reginald Bosanquet (anchorman), Astronaut Jim Irwin and GS.

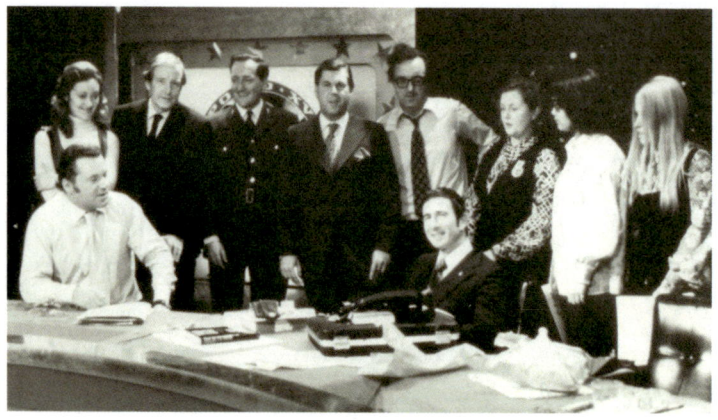

The ITN Special Space Programmes team. Standing left to right: Valerie Morrison, Frank Miles, GS, Peter Fairley, David Nicholas, Diana Edwards-Jones, Christine Lomas, Carole de Caux. Seated: Reginald Bosanquet and Jim

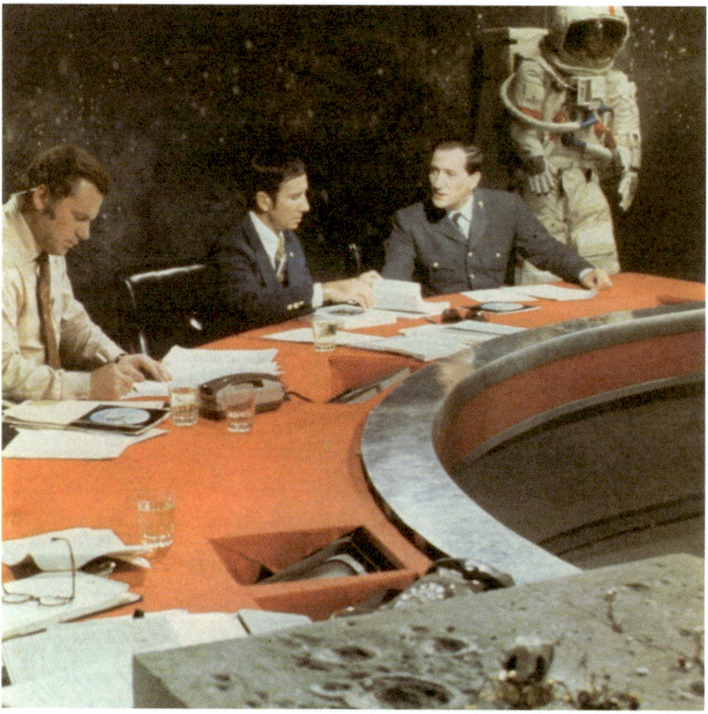

Talking to Jim Irwin and Reginald Bosanquet in the studio of ITN during the Apollo 17 mission.

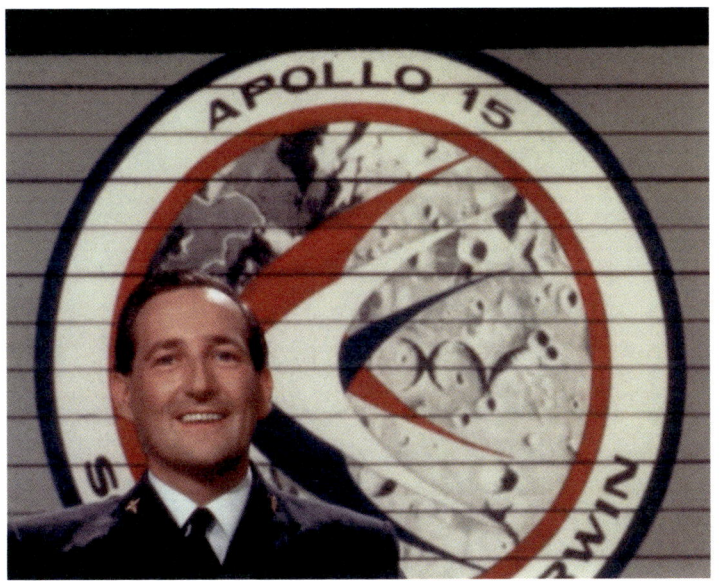

On air during the Apollo 15 mission

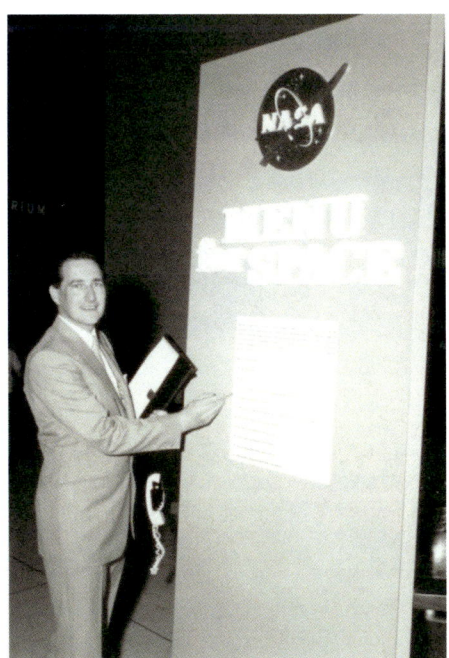

Preparing for a broadcast by satellite from the Manned Spacecraft Centre, Houston, to ITN House in London. Topic – food in space.

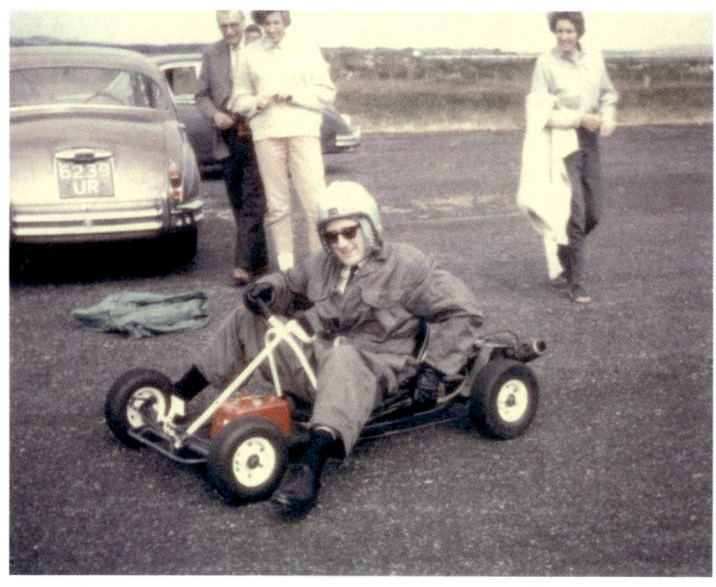

Testing out an early kart on the runway of the old airfield at Evanton.

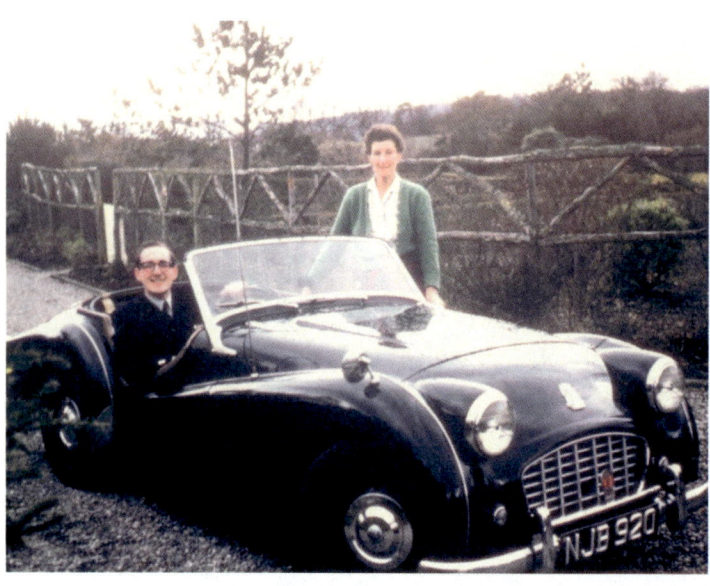

In my Triumph TR2, Mother looking on.

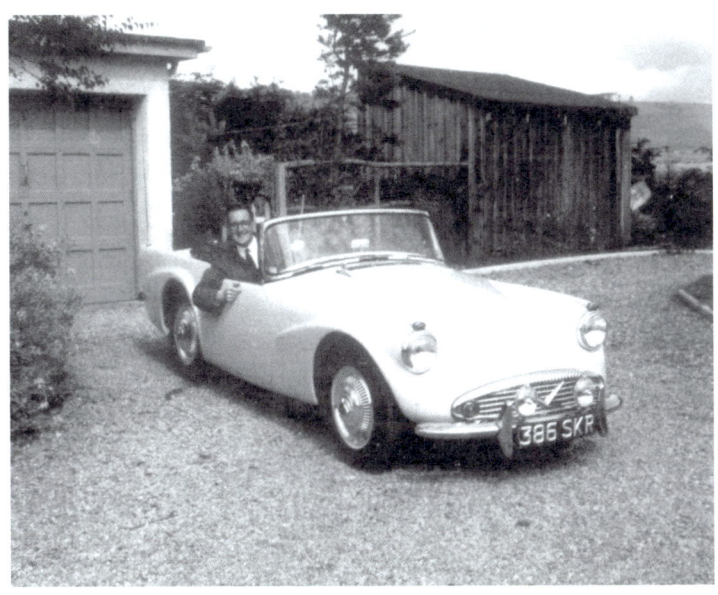

The yellow Daimler SP250 which had belonged to Val Parnell

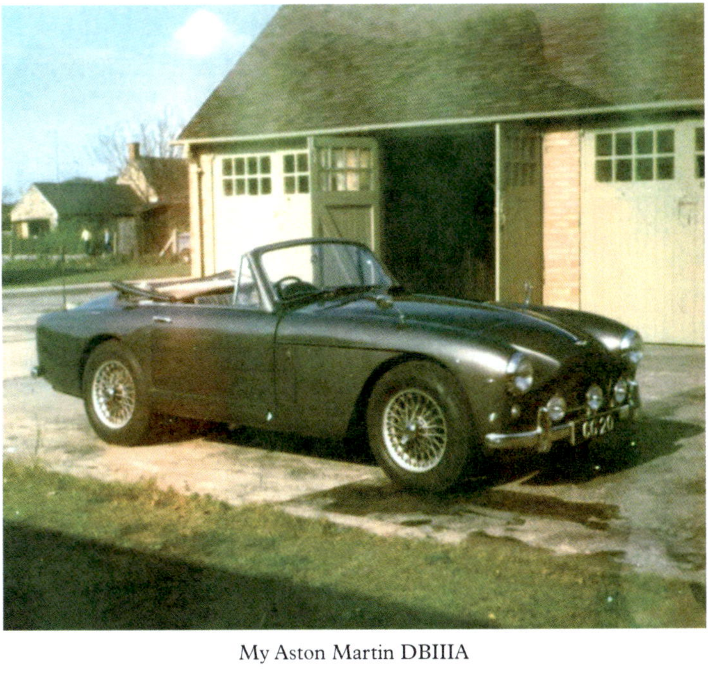

My Aston Martin DBIIIA

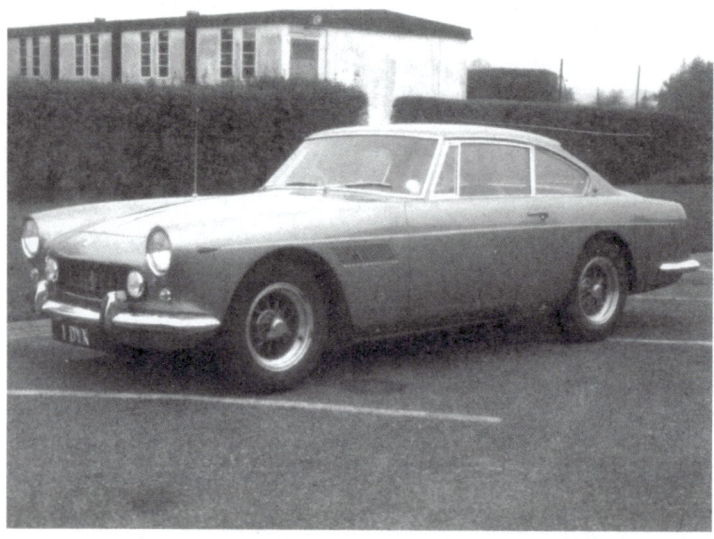

The Ferrari 250 GT/E, formerly Dickie Henderson's pride and joy

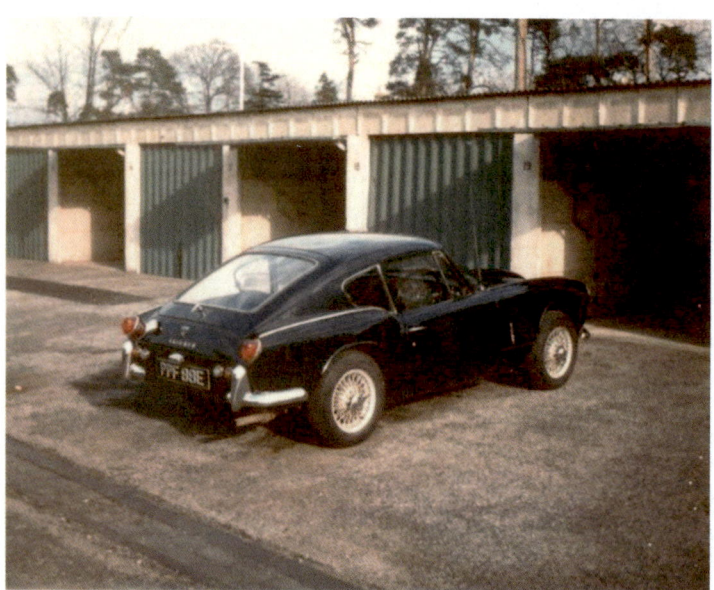

My Triumph GT6

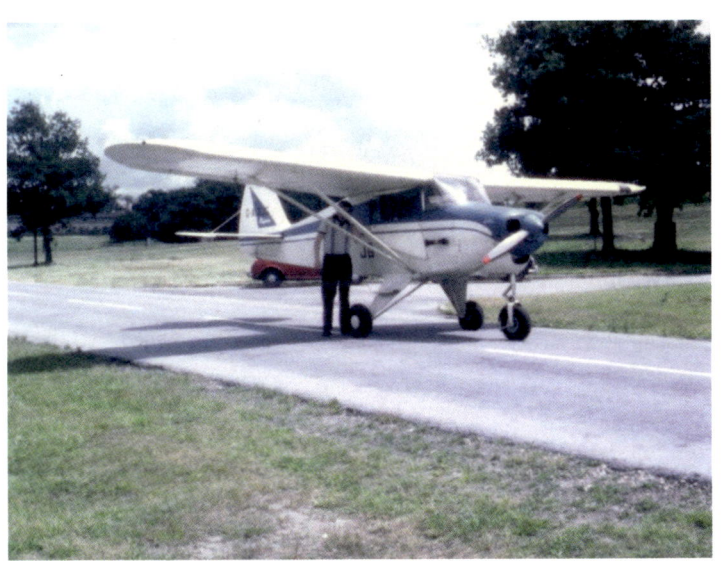
My Piper Colt, 'Julie Golf'

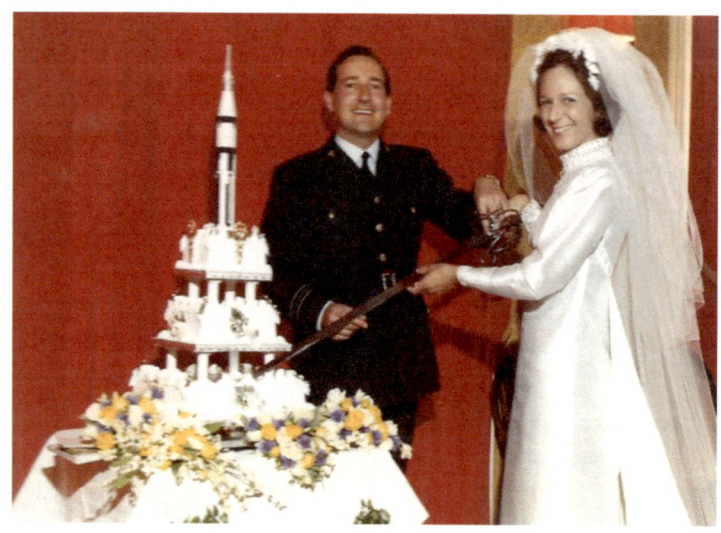

Our wedding day, August 19 1972. The cake was topped by an atlas rocket!

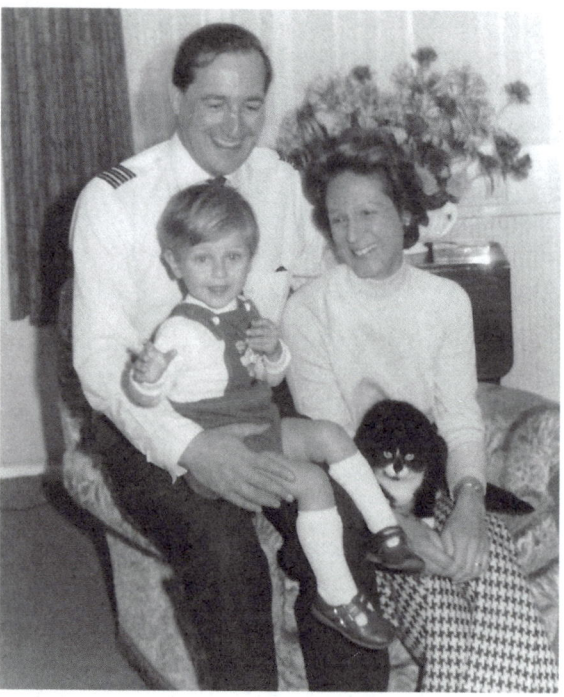

At North Luffenham in the early days, Russell aged about two

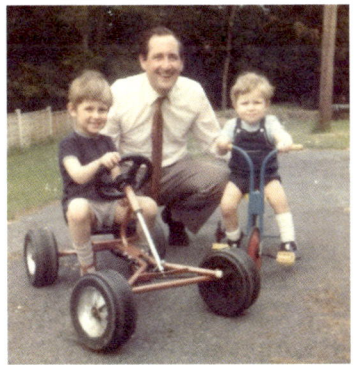

The boys with me in Farnham, 1979, Russell on four wheels and Willie on three

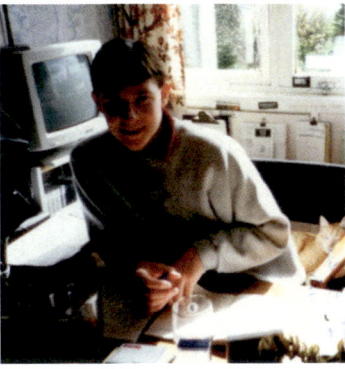

Willie at home – he was obsessed with flying and turned his bedroom into an air traffic control centre.

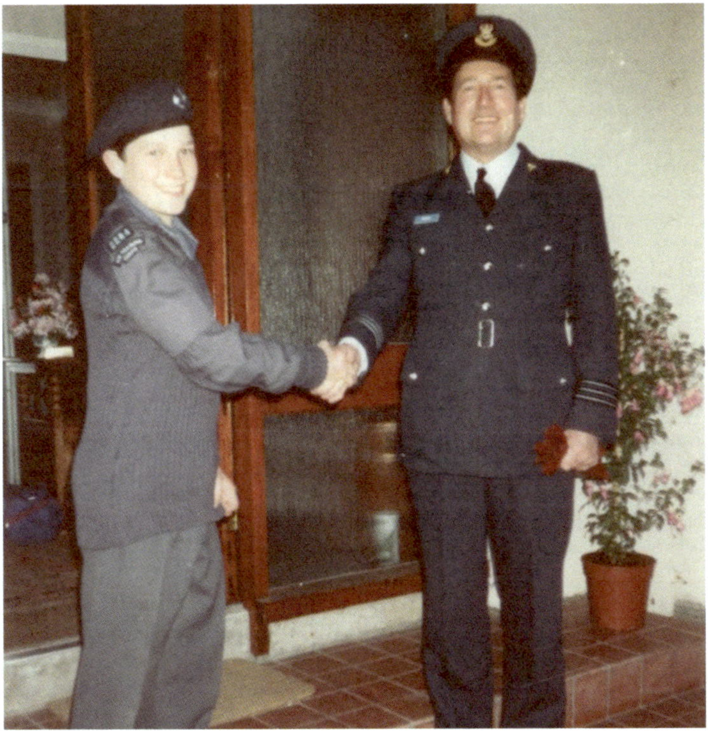

Shaking hands with my second son Willie, both of us in RAF uniform, when he was a young cadet in Dunblane air cadets. I had just reviewed them on their annual parade.

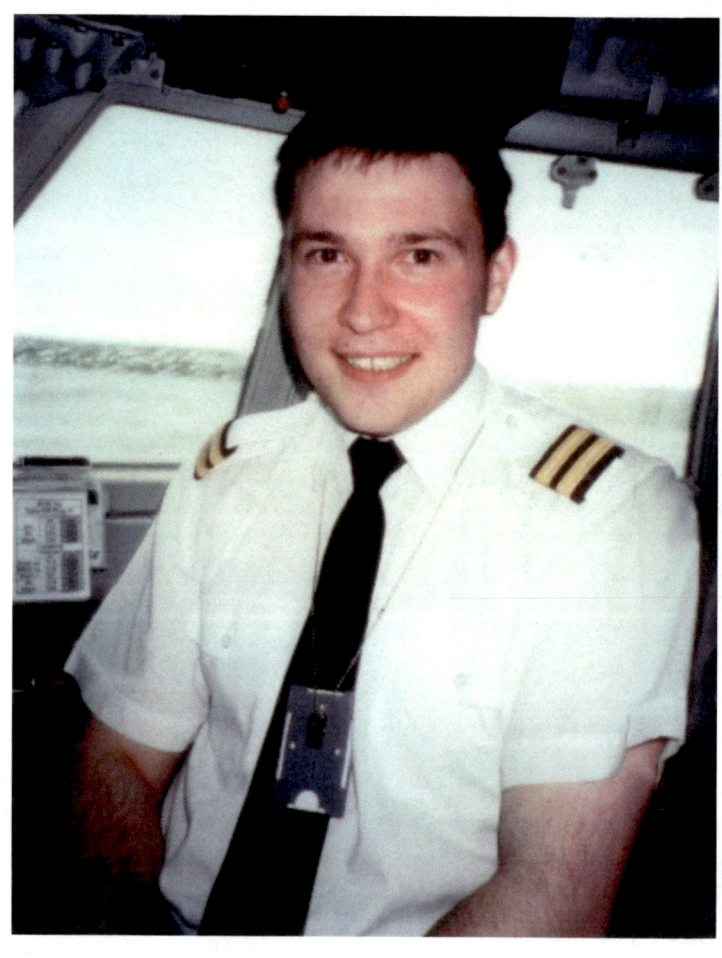

Willie in the cockpit on becoming a First Officer for
British Regional Airways and later Britannia Airways.

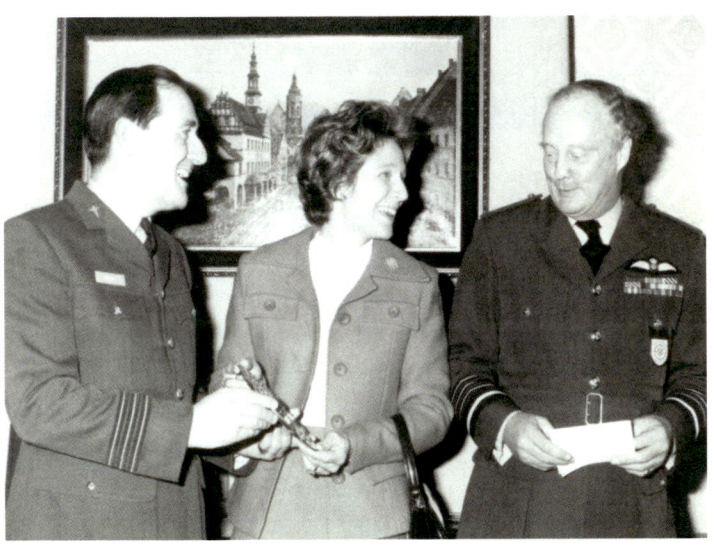

With Kirstie at the presentation of the Richard Fox Linton Award in 1976 by Air Chief Marshal Sir Nigel Maynard.

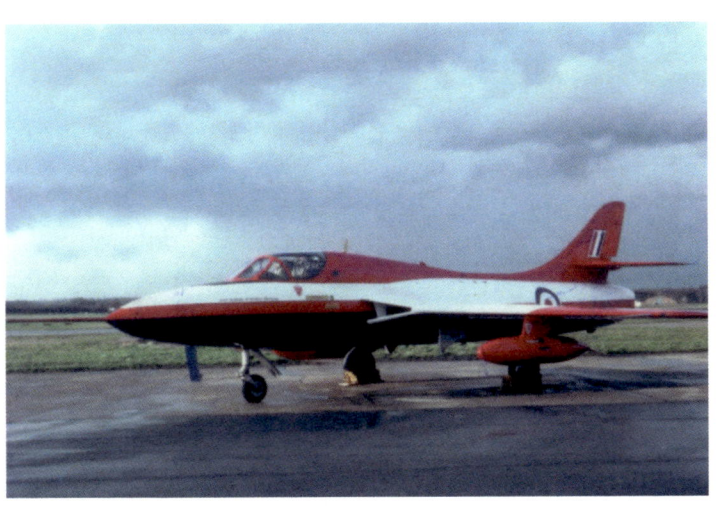

The Institute's Hunter T4. Much of the in-flight work was carried out in this and our Canberra bomber.

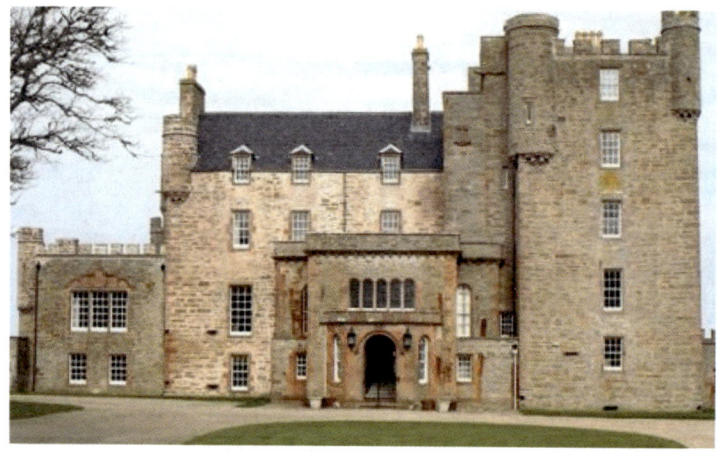

The Castle of Mey front entrance, used only by the Queen Mother. Staff used the Courtyard entrance.

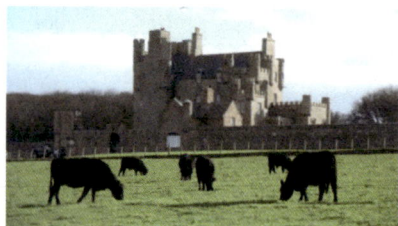

Another view of the Castle of Mey showing the QM's beloved prize cattle in the foreground.

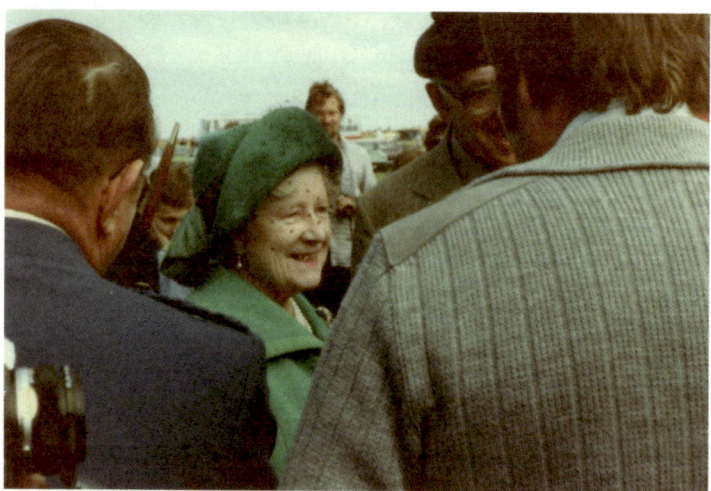

Kirstie's own photo of the Queen Mother taken during her annual Mey Games. She is talking to some of the organisers.

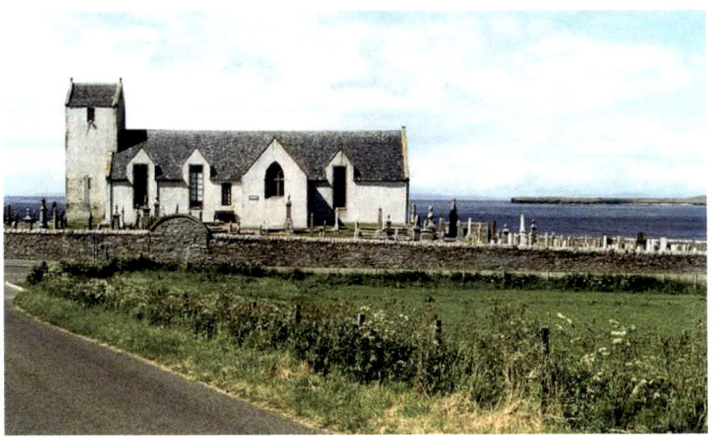

Canisbay Church, where the Queen Mother worshipped during her visits to the Castle of Mey.

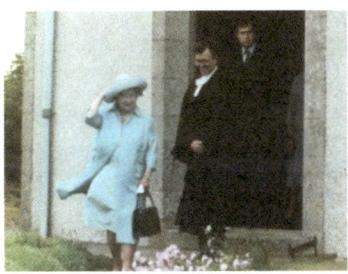

The QM with Reverend Alec Muir, leaving Canisbay Church.

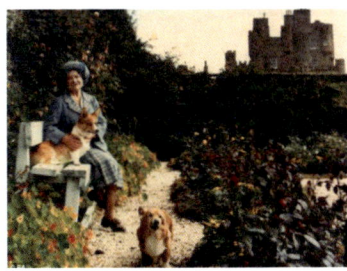

The Queen Mother in the 'Policies', seated by the Shell Garden, one of her favourite spots.

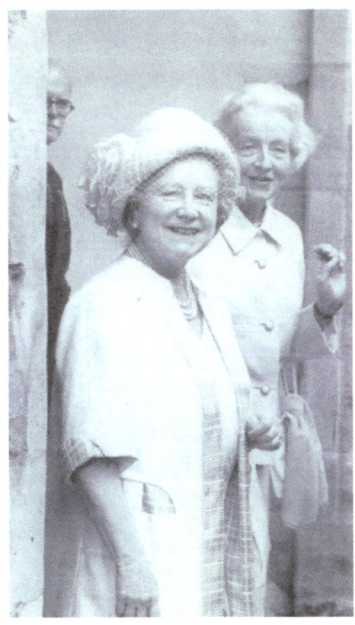

A newspaper photo of the QM with Ruth, Lady Fermoy, who helped me care for a guest who had collapsed at the Castle (Eastern Daily Press).

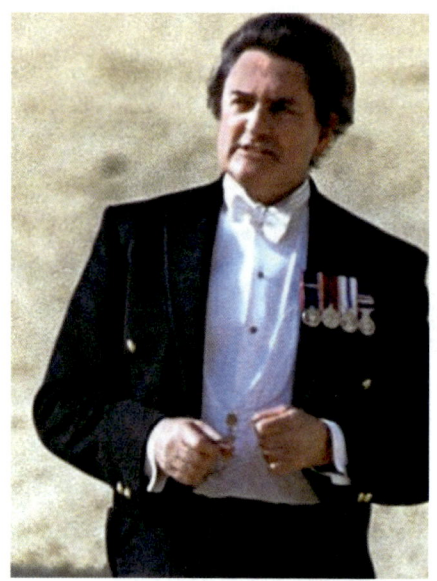

William Tallon, the Queen Mother's personal page - known to all as 'Backstairs Billy'.

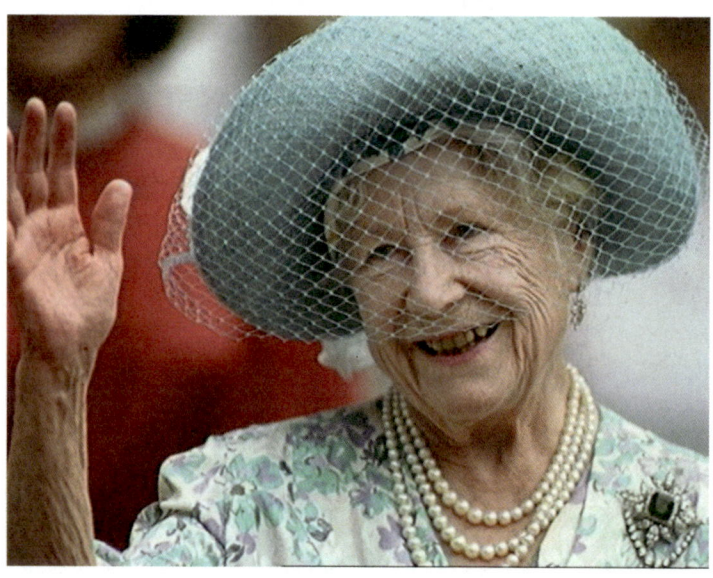

The Queen Mother as everyone remembers her

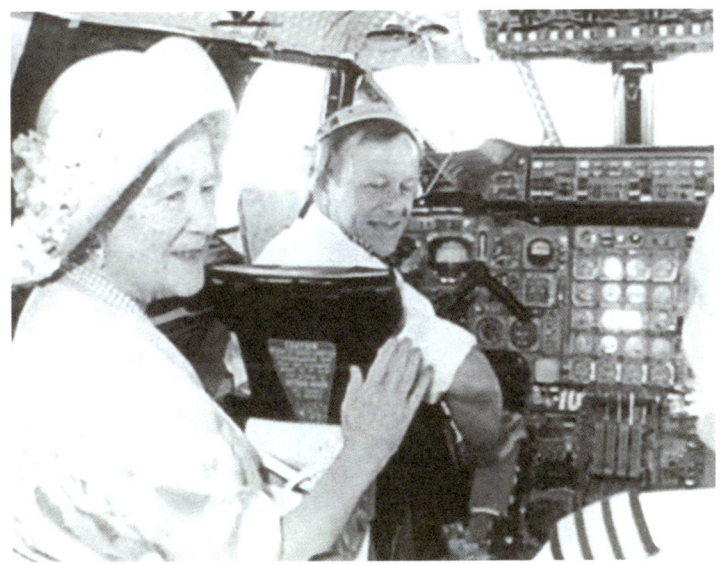

The QM fulfils her dream of a flight on Concorde

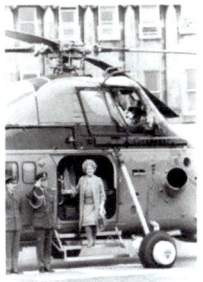

Her Majesty loved helicopters!

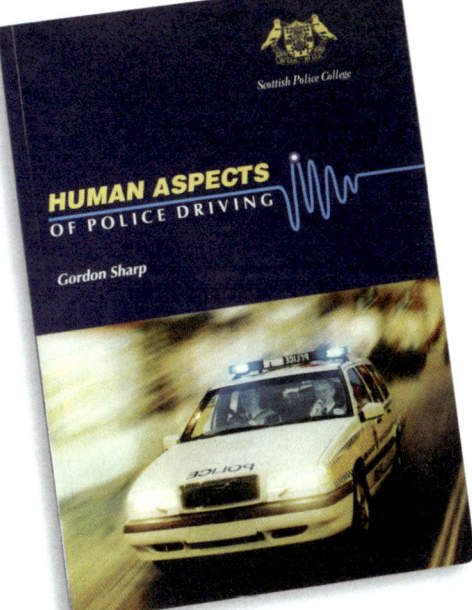

My book Human Aspects of Police Driving, written with the support of the Scottish police.

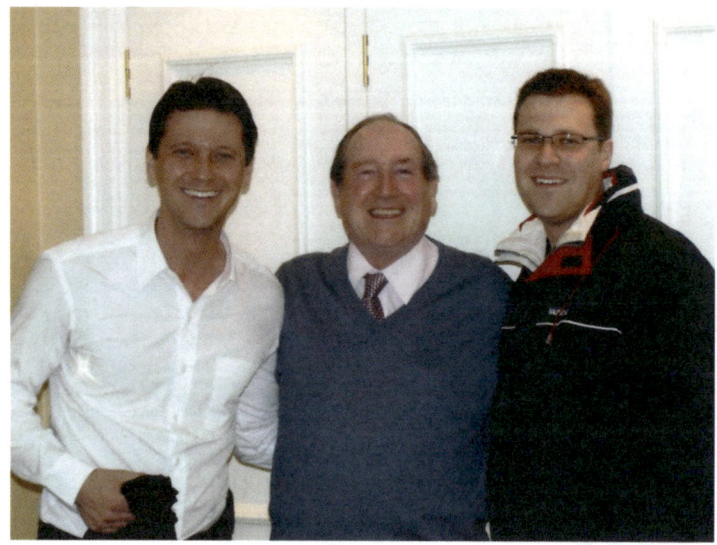

With Russell and Alastair at my 75th birthday celebration at the Grosvenor House Hotel, April 2010.

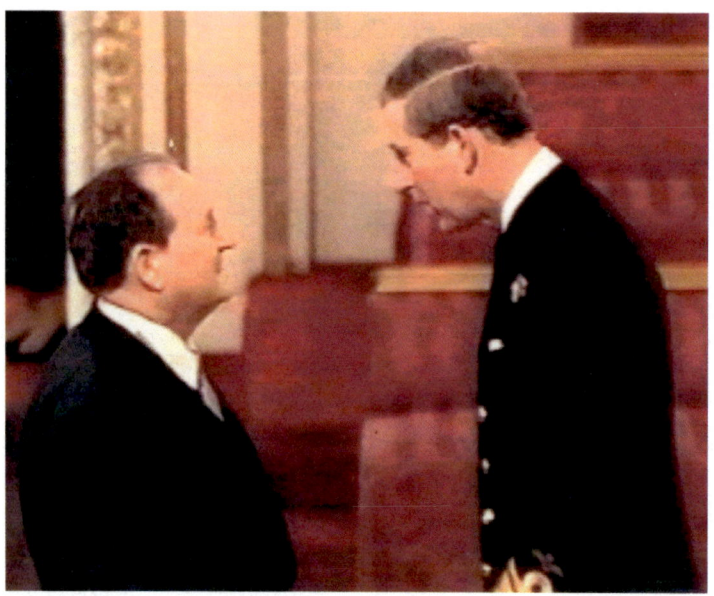

HRH Prince Charles presents my MBE at Buckingham Palace.

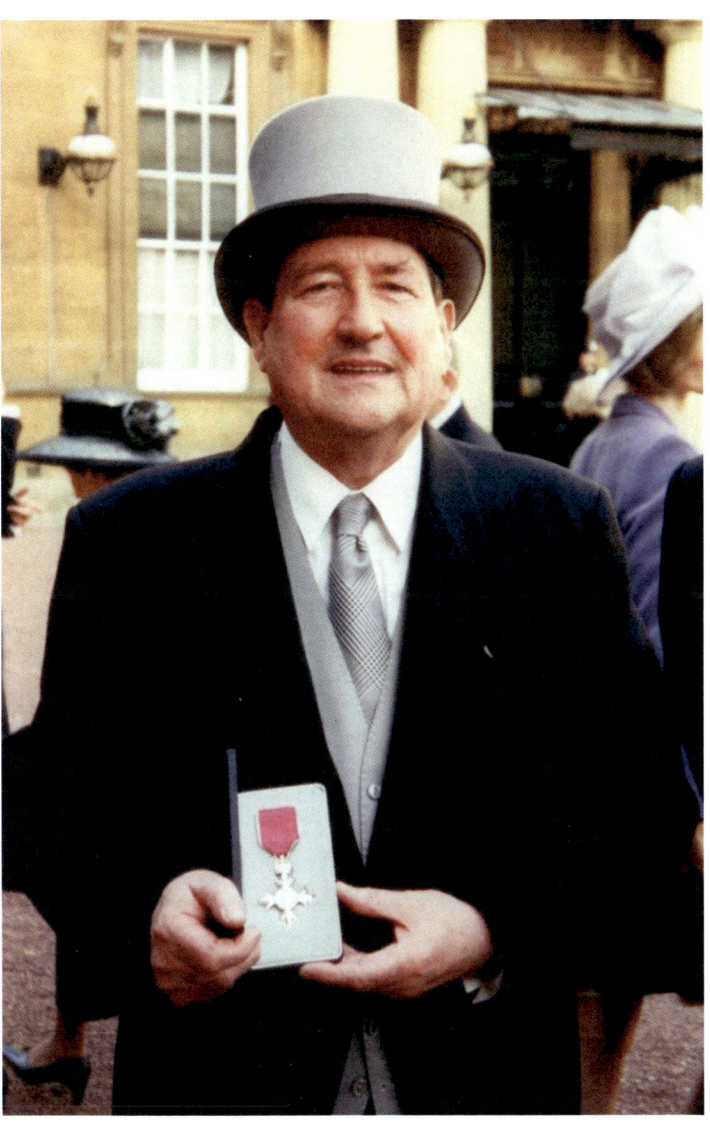

Proudly clutching my unexpected honour.

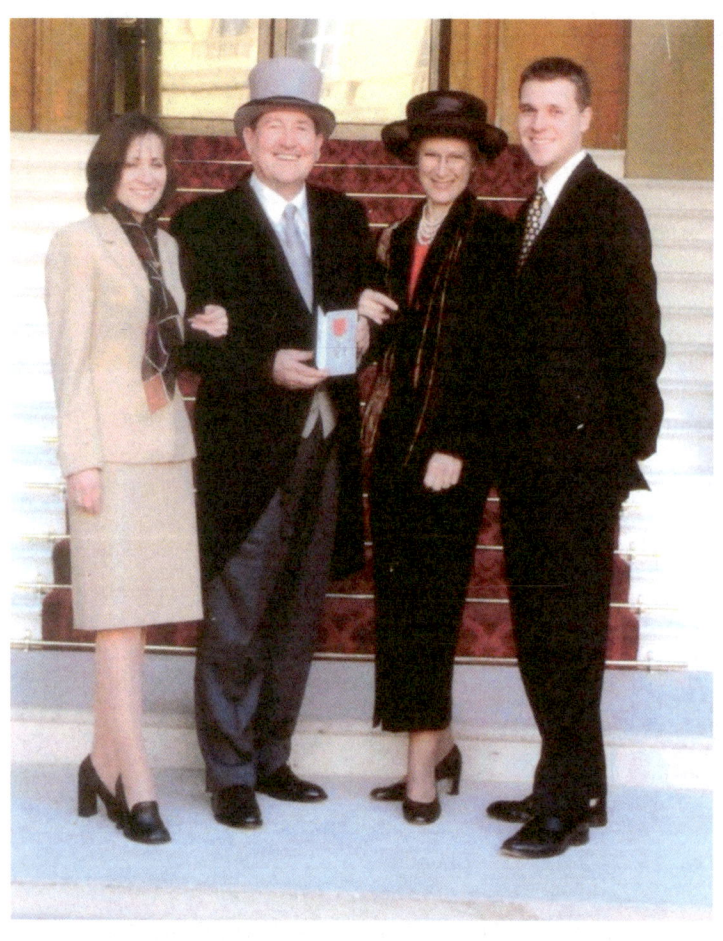

On the steps of Buckingham Palace after the investiture with Melanie, Kirstie and Alastair.

CHAPTER SIX

A CHANGE IN THE WIND

I returned to the UK in time to celebrate Christmas, and it was quite a shock to be plunged into a British winter. It contrasted greatly with the carol-singing and pulling of crackers the previous Christmas in the desert, in a temperature of 96 degrees. I was a little shocked by the cold after my two years in the Middle East, but I was very pleased to be back on familiar territory, in more senses than one. It was good to get back into the social whirl again and catch up with the social scene in Scotland.

My time out in the Middle East had certainly not been wasted. I had made many friends and gained new and valuable experiences. I had enjoyed my first real taste of

being at the 'sharp end' of military operational flying and had taken every opportunity to get my hands on as many aircraft as I could and fly them if possible.

Perhaps most important of all, my experiences had taught

me that I didn't need the massively expensive capital equipment I had used at IAM to do useful scientific work. It confirmed that the most useful equipment of all was what the RAF called the 'Mark 1 Eyeball' – simple observations which led in many cases to discoveries that would help to make aviation safer for pilots.

I thought long and hard about the possibility that I might make this type of applied field study my own special area of aviation medicine research. This was something for the future, and I tucked the thought away to the back of my mind. Now there was exciting work to do, and my aviation medicine career was about to begin. This would be my stepping stone back to the Mecca of all aviation medicine research - IAM Farnborough.

I took up my new posting at the Aeromedical Training Centre or AMTC (as it was then called), which had been set up a few years previously at RAF Upwood in Cambridgeshire to centralise the training of aircrew in the protective clothing and assemblies needed to protect them in high altitude flight. They were trained how to cope with in-flight emergencies and given practical demonstrations and experience of sudden loss of cabin pressure at high altitude in one of the Centre's decompression chambers.

John Ernsting had supervised the setting up of the Unit, but it soon became clear to him that the facilities and the small team of non-specialist doctors could not easily keep up with the rapid advances in military operations and the complexities of new aircraft soon to come into service. He was now looking to increase the number of staff, extend the scope of training and seek more suitable accommodation to house the extended training facilities needed for the future.

We were to form the core of that new unit. The newly-appointed CO was Wing Commander Tom Dobie, who had been a pilot before he took up medicine. He was a ball of fire, always full of energy and getting things done. A good-natured man, he became my good friend and drinking companion. Tom had asked the Air Ministry to give him Medical Officers with aviation medicine and physiology experience, and I and another MO, plus two other general medical officers, made up his new team.

Upwood had been a former wartime bomber station and we shared it with the RAF regiment, although we never saw much of their activities. Much of their time seemed to be spent running round the airfield perimeter carrying a heavy wooden telephone pole. Even then their efforts were masked by a constant morning fog which regularly drifted in from the Fens and enveloped the airfield for much of the day. I did not take to that Station, but I took heart from the fact that I would be putting to good use the research work I had carried out at IAM with Pete Wagner.

It was at Upwood that I first met Donald Cameron, who was to become a lifelong friend. Like me, Don was desperate to get into the IAM and had courageously given up his GP practice in Doncaster. He had graduated the previous year with a BSc in physiology from Edinburgh University with the promise that if he joined the RAF there might be a chance to fulfil his dreams. He was a qualified civilian pilot and part-time flying instructor, so he brought a welcome skill to the newly-formed team. It wasn't long before he and I were made Specialists in Aviation Medicine, and with the other members we set about radically altering the AMTC.

The first priority was to find suitable accommodation in

which we could house three mobile decompression chambers, which were crucial to the final and most important part of the training - to give the aircrew confidence in their equipment and put them through the rapid decompression which would simulate the actual emergency of an inflight loss of cabin pressure. It was also the most dangerous part of the training, and Tom Dobie and the rest of the team were worried that the cramped and restricted facilities at Upwood were inadequate to allow us to monitor the wellbeing and safety of crew undergoing the RD experience. Tom set about looking for possible new accommodation and the rest of the team began revamping teaching notes, lectures and training procedures.

Tom came in full of excitement one morning to tell us that he had found the perfect site for our new centre. It was at RAF North Luffenham, close to the village of Edith Weston, a few miles up the A1 from us. It had been home to a former Royal Canadian Air Force fighter Squadron and had more recently been occupied by one of the UK bases for the Thor intermediate range ballistic missiles. The personnel, largely Americans, who had manned the base had uplifted the Thor missiles in a massive USAF freighter aircraft and left for the States. The station was now up for grabs, and Tom, spotting the ideal site for our new unit, had put in a successful bid to the Ministry of Defence.

He enthused that it would provide excellent accommodation for visiting aircrew courses, and with a little modification one of the buildings would be ideal for training and equipping the aircrew. His announcement that we would be moving to a new base was greeted with less than enthusiasm. However, when he told them that the outgoing Americans had left behind a magnificent ten-pin bowling alley and enough crates of bourbon and whisky liqueur (Southern Comfort) to last for many years, attitudes and enthusiasm for the move changed dramatically.

After weeks of preparation packing and sorting out all our equipment, we made the move up the A1 over the Easter Holiday weekend; all leave was cancelled. It must have been quite a remarkable sight for the local residents, who had only recently watched the uplift of the massive Thor missiles. Now they were witnessing convoys of RAF lorries and large tractor vehicles towing our decompression chambers and their pump trailers trundling through their villages. It was an exhausting weekend for us all, but the airmen and NCOs in our team worked their socks off and we were ready for the first course of aircrew in time for the following Tuesday. It was quite an achievement.

Once settled into our new premises, we needed to address the next important problem. It was becoming of increasing concern that during the training runs in our decompression chambers some of the pilots were collapsing from a type of vasovagal faint. This was a potentially disastrous problem for obvious reasons, and one that threatened to destroy all confidence in the protection given by their oxygen equipment and assemblies in the event of an emergency. This had to be addressed urgently, so we reviewed the techniques of monitoring the body systems during the practical training and the rapid decompression runs. We improved the monitoring of heart rate and rhythm during the rapid decompression and I developed a training aid - a small device which would measure breathing rates and volumes of the pilot in the chamber.

Despite these efforts we were still getting an unacceptable

number of collapses. It was then that I took it upon myself to adapt one of the tricks used by test pilots evaluating a new aircraft. I looked for any variation on the established and well-tested training procedures which might give a clue to the cause of the problem. It had worked for me in Bahrain, and I was sure it could work again for me now.

The difference turned out to be that on the last evening of the course, aircrew met up in the Mess bar and celebrated in style. They came in the next morning (the day of the rapid decompression experience) with mild hangovers. Under normal circumstances this would be of little consequence, but with the demands of the training on the body systems even a mild hangover could tip them over into a vasovagal collapse situation (similar to a fainting attack). When I suggested that it was probably the beer consumption that was causing the problem, hands went up in horror!

I was warned that we had to handle this one very carefully as the excellent and popular local brew was Ruddles' beer and Sir Kenneth Ruddle, the founder and owner of the brewery, was a highly-respected and long-standing honorary member of the Mess.

Faced with this problem, I suggested that we might resort to an approach that had been successful in dealing with injury problems in parachutists in Bahrain - if you can't get round a major operational problem, try to make a simple rearrangement of routine or procedures. This approach had taken care of a landing hazard and reduced the number of injuries.

Taking the same approach, I rearranged the course programme, bringing the rapid decompression experience forward to an earlier point in the training. This simple change put a stop to the end-of-course parties and the excessive beer consumption. Recalling the 'farting experiments' I had participated in at IAM, I also suggested the further precaution of avoiding gas-producing foods on the night before the rapid decompressions. After that there was a huge reduction in the number of collapses, at least collapses in the decompression chamber! It strengthened my belief in the policy of looking for simple explanations of problems first, and using equally simple and minimally disruptive measures to put things right.

It was not long before my passion for cars was rekindled. I had been on the lookout for a Jaguar XK120, but one day in 1964 I spotted a daffodil yellow Daimler SP250 in a showroom off Bond Street in London and fell for it. It had belonged to Val Parnell, the theatrical impresario and the TV producer behind *Sunday Night at the London Palladium*, and had been used by Bernard Delfont, an equally famous impresario. I fell for that car and bought it on the spot. It was a two-seater open sports car (formerly known as the Daimler Dart, until Chrysler threatened legal action over use of the name) and had a V8 2.5 litre engine which took it to around 120 miles per hour, a fast car for those days.

The Daimler played an important part in my social life. Around this time I began to meet up with a lovely girl called Heather. I knew her from way back in the days of our early teens, when our two families had met up every year for a fortnight's holiday at the Marine Hotel in Rosemarkie on the Black Isle in Scotland. These were the days when family holidays were in vogue, and Heather was the great attraction of the day. She was an excellent dancer and good at sports.

We rather lost touch when I left University, but when I heard that she was in London I got in contact with her straight away.

We spent a lot of time together in London after that, mainly at the weekends. I would motor down from North Luffenham and stay at the RAF club. We often dined at Chez Auguste, a delightful French restaurant in Soho, taking in a show, a film or a visit to a night club. She was working for the BBC and living in Holland Park. I became very keen on Heather, and was beginning to see her as a possible partner for life. I had even picked out a suitable engagement ring from a jewellers in the Burlington Arcade.

But it was not to be. Heather was never free to see me in the week and I began to suspect there might be someone else on the scene. In the end I discovered that she had fallen for a South African chap who had bowled her off her feet. Unlike me, he was able to spend all his time with her, so she chose him. I entirely understood her situation, but I was very upset at the time.

To add to my gloom that year, my father was suddenly taken ill with a heart attack. He died on December 18 1964, aged only 64, before I had had a chance to say goodbye. He had been quite a heavy smoker, but I have a feeling he died of boredom, having given up a very active business life for the less stimulating routine of retirement. Naturally I missed him terribly, and was concerned about how Mum would cope with the future as a widow.

I needn't have worried. In her typical practical manner she set about involving herself in every possible committee and club activity. This helped her to overcome her loss, and it was a great relief to me that she was coping so well.

After a while I sold the Daimler, largely because of the

association with Heather. The whiff of her expensive perfume still hung around the inside of the car, a constant lingering reminder of her. I swapped it for an Aston Martin DBIIIA, a wonderful car and a highlight of my motoring career. It turned out that it had an experimental engine, built, I believe, as a prototype for the later Vantage engine. It sounded like a cement mixer when you started it up, but once the engine was warmed up it emitted the most magnificent growl and went like stink. It drew a great deal of attention on visits to the US Air Force Officers' Club at Alconbury and I had several offers for it.

One day I noticed that an unsightly round mark had appeared on the bodywork. The David Brown factory at Newport Pagnell wasn't far away, so I drove it along there and showed it to them. They said they knew what the problem was and it would all be taken care of, and I was invited to have a cup of coffee while I waited. From the chassis number they identified the exact paint which had been used – not just the same colour but the actual paint – and went to work. Within no time at all it was as good as new.

While I was waiting for my car to be returned I was interested to be shown an early and very rare Lionel Martin LM2 which was being treated as a precautionary measure for woodworm in some of its body hoops, of all things.

The real treat came when I discovered that they had the very DB5 model which had been used in the James Bond film *Goldfinger*. I was thrilled to see the car and inspect it in the workshop, and even more delighted when the workshop manager offered to take me for a short spin in it. What a thrilling experience it was. Although I knew it was based on a standard model, I was fascinated by the dummy guns and the spinning knives on the wheels. Fortunately the ejector seat was a dummy too, otherwise my life and career might have been brought to a sudden end.

I continued to run the Aston for some time during my tour at North Luffenham, and quite enjoyed the attention it received in the car park of our local pub at Wing. That is, until one evening David Brown himself arrived in a unique Lagonda - an absolute beauty, with every conceivable luxury and piece of built-in gadgetry you could imagine. It had been made to his own design, a one-off model specially built for him in his own factory. You couldn't get near it for people inspecting it and drooling over its beautiful lines. It made my poor little Aston look positively shabby sitting alongside it.

Shortly after that I took the Aston down to RAF Biggin Hill, where the AMTC was putting on an exhibition display stand showing the work of the Centre. It was held in a large hangar close to the main runway and dispersal area used by the Battle of Britain Spitfire Squadrons during World War 2, next door to a similar hangar in which Tom Dobie had spotted a wartime German bomber - a Junkers Ju88. Although entry to the aircraft was forbidden, Tom, with his insatiable curiosity, had managed to find someone who held the key, and he asked me to join him for an inspection of the inside of the bomber.

It was amazing to sit up in the pilot's seat with its all-round view, and I found it a very evocative experience to take up the bomb-aimer's position. Looking down at the floor of the hangar I couldn't but wonder if that aircraft might just have been the very one that had destroyed our house and changed my life on the night of the Clydebank Blitz. I gave a shudder at the thought and began to extricate myself from the bomb aimer's cramped position.

When I rejoined my colleagues on the exhibition stand, I realised that the keys to my Aston were no longer in my pocket. My heart sank.

'Don't panic' said the ever-calm Tom Dobie. 'You nip back to the hangar and see if you dropped them in the Junkers or on the hangar floor. I'll go to the garage in the village and see if we can get some help.'

After a long and frantic search I found the keys just as Tom had predicted, lying on the floor of the Junkers. When Tom returned he too was relieved, as he had had no luck in finding assistance. What he had found, however, was something quite special. He had spotted in the garage showroom a silver-grey Ferrari which he thought would be just perfect for me, with my love of classic cars.

The car he had spotted was a 250GT/E which I believe had belonged to the entertainer Dickie Henderson and still bore the registration plate 1 DYX. That was a stunning car and a spectacular performer, with a 240 bhp V6 engine and a separate carburettor for each cylinder. Today it would be worth a fortune, particularly with that plate on it. I was able to buy it almost as a straight swap.

Unfortunately it attracted even more attention back at the base than the Aston, and they all wanted to sit in it. One chap climbed in, let out the clutch and promptly shot backwards into the Station Commander's favourite rose bed. I was not very popular with Station HQ after that.

I greatly enjoyed driving that Ferrari, and its performance was quite literally breathtaking. The acceleration was amazing, and so powerful was the torque from the engine that when I pressed the accelerator pedal I was thrust backwards with a thump into the driving seat. One snag was that it was a swine to keep the six carburettors in tune and the car was in and out of the late racing driver Mike Hawthorn's garage in Farnham like a yo-yo. I used the opportunity of every visit to Farnborough to get the Ferrari-trained mechanics to balance them.

Unfortunately I damaged the exhaust pipe on it, which proved to be an expensive mistake. The exhaust systems on these cars were built and tuned by Abarth in Italy and replacing them cost a king's ransom. I took it as usual to Mike Hawthorn's garage and they managed to adapt the pipe from a lorry exhaust, but although it was an effective repair the mechanics gloomily predicted that the car would never quite be the same after that. They went into great explanation of how the repair had probably altered the impedance of the whole Abarth exhaust system and the engine wouldn't like that. To my mind, however, there seemed to be no change in the speed and acceleration and its performance still frightened me fartless when I put my foot down on the accelerator.

A new Medical Officer, Flight Lieutenant Mike Henderson, then joined our team. He had a passion for racing cars and a longing to improve safety in motor sport. During his time at AMTC he of course took great interest in the Ferrari and often took it for a spin through the narrow roads of the Rutland countryside, always at top speed, I suspect. I don't know how much influence my car had on his interest, but while he was with us he wrote an excellent book called *Motor Racing in Safety*. Mike later went to Australia and became Chairman of the Australian Institute for Motor Sport. From there he introduced the six-point harness, which became a standard requirement in international motor racing. He was a brilliant doctor, physiologist and amateur racing driver and I often wondered if the experience of being thumped back in the seat of my Ferrari influenced the final design of his seat harness!

We were now just beginning to enjoy the fruits of our hard work at the AMTC, and there was a much more relaxed atmosphere among visiting aircrew, who no longer dreaded the experience in the decompression chamber. One morning Tom Dobie asked me into his office and started talking about all the achievements of the team and how the prestige of the Centre had been lifted in the eyes of the Ministry of Defence. It was unusual for Tom to talk like this, and I couldn't help thinking that there must be an ulterior motive to his conversation. What project was he cooking up now, and what was he going to involve me in?

'How would you like to go out to Cyprus and give the pilots of the Iraqi Air Force some training in aviation medicine?' he said, straight out.

'The Iraqi Air Force?' I spluttered in astonishment. 'What on earth is going on?'

'I don't know much about it, but basically the Iraqis are looking to purchase some British aircraft to supplement their squadrons of Russian-built Mig 15 and 21 aircraft' he explained. 'They don't seem to like the Soviet Michelin Man flying gear the Russians have left them with, it's too bulky. They know nothing about how our guys' protective kit works in an explosive decompression and they haven't a clue about our oxygen systems, pressure breathing or anything else. The Director of Medical Services wants you to meet about a dozen of their senior pilots in RAF Akrotiri and try and push hard all the advantages of our aircraft and our life-support systems. It should take about three weeks, they reckon. It'll give you the opportunity to get your knees brown again!'

'God almighty, is that all MoD want me to do?' I said sarcastically. I had about a thousand questions to ask, but Tom went on to say, 'You'll be using the Mobile Chamber at RAF Akrotiri and I've arranged for one of our corporal chamber operators to accompany you. Best of luck, you're off there in five days' time.'

I had been looking forward to a week or two on the beautiful island of Cyprus, but any thoughts that it was going to be a holiday were shattered when the training started. Although most of them had a reasonable understanding of English, it took all my skills at teaching and training to demonstrate the advantages of our RAF system.

When I eventually got them ready to go into the decompression chamber, a few pilots had difficulty in coping with the unusual sensation of a tight chest when the oxygen system delivered pressure at simulated altitude. They pulled off their masks, and we had to crash the chamber to ground level on frequent occasions. Monitoring was difficult because we didn't have the equipment we had at Luffenham and they couldn't communicate easily without the aid of an interpreter (who of course couldn't be in the chamber with them). They did their best using hand gestures, but the corporal technician was beside himself with worry at not being able to spot when they were in difficulty.

'What do I do when all they can do is testiculate?' he pleaded. By which he meant they threw their arms about and talked a lot of balls into the microphone!

Somehow we managed to get to the end of the training in

one piece, and the pilots all seemed to be very happy with what they had learned. Through their interpreter I learned that they all considered the meeting a huge success - all the pressure breathing problems seemed to have been forgotten.

During their visit they managed to clean out the NAAFI stocks of children's clothing and other goods to take home. The NAAFI Manager was far from pleased, but he had just about got over his displeasure when we waved them off in their C130 aircraft back to Baghdad. As their aircraft became a dot in the sky and they headed for home I sighed with relief and relished the thought that I would now be able to enjoy some time in the sun and the pleasures which Cyprus had to offer.

Unfortunately there was one more little problem to deal with before the adventure was over. The duty officer phoned to say that the Iraqi officers were on their way back to Cyprus; the catering staff had provided an in-flight snack of ham sandwiches! When they opened their meal pack and found them, the captain of the aircraft refused to land in Baghdad with the forbidden pig meat. The catering staff were very red-faced about their blunder and fixed them up with an alternative, which seemed to go down well. So international relations were saved and I hoped that I had fulfilled my duty of promoting British aircraft and our life support equipment.

After that the remaining week of my detachment did indeed become one of leisure and exploring the beautiful island of Cyprus. It was then that I met Flying Officer 'Chalky' White, a zany character if ever there was one. Chalky was known as 'chameleon', apparently because he was brilliant at avoiding capture during the escape and evasion exercises which were held in RAF Germany at that time. He told me the secret of his ability to outwit the German police, who were always roped in to seek out and 'capture' the course members and take them in for 'interrogation' - not always a pleasant one, it has to be said. One of the instructors whom he met in a pub quoted an old German expression which went, '*Nur tote Fische schwimmen mit dem Strom*', which literally translates as 'only dead fish swim with the stream'. He meant 'think for yourself rather than unquestioningly follow the group'.

Chalky put this advice to good use during the escape and evasion exercise. At the start of the exercise he remained close to the dropping-off point, climbing up a tree and 'making like a chameleon', as he put it. From there he watched the German police volunteers pick up the other course members one by one. They had all gone with the herd. The 'searchers' knew exactly where they would go, and it was easy to follow their tracks in the snow. Chalky remained up his tree until the search was called off and the exercise came to an end. The German police, with all their thoroughness and experience, simply couldn't understand how they had been hoodwinked by this man. Chalky had learned that sometimes taking the unusual and unexpected pathway and not simply following the herd can often pay off. That was a lesson to remember.

He also introduced me to the delights of the Cypriot brandy shops, and he and his wife were very hospitable and showed me the sights of the island. He remained a good friend, and I visited the family back in UK when their tour ended.

On my return to North Luffenham and the Centre, the difficulties in communication which had been such a problem in training the Iraqis in Cyprus were still in my mind. If only we had been able to lay on demonstrations or give the pilots a picture of what was to come in the chamber, things would have been easier. I was still looking at ways in which we could improve our training and demonstrating at AMTC and what lessons I could learn from that experience. I felt there was something missing, and tried to work out what it could be.

It was then that I resurrected my boyhood interest in broadcasting and wondered if I had found the answer. Curiously enough, my father often told me of his training days in the Research Division at Metrovick in Manchester, and how he had been involved in the launch of BBC Radio Manchester. Trainees helped out by setting up microphones and operating switchgear in their makeshift studio. As often as not he was called upon to help in programmes like 'Children's Corner', where each of the trainees would take turns at playing 'Uncle Humpty Dumpty'. They made up ad-lib programmes and Dad told me how difficult he found it to make talks on gardening and even welding sound interesting.

I then recalled that as a young lad I too had spent many happy hours tinkering with microphones (I remember buying one from a war surplus shop) and connecting them to my parents' old Ferguson wireless set. Like Dad before me, I started to make up my own little programmes from my bedroom (my parents in the lounge downstairs were the only audience). I read and acted stories, poems and sang songs, complete with animal noises and various sound effects trying to add interest to my amateur 'broadcast'. Full of self-confidence, I even wrote to Kathleen Garscadden ('Aunty Kathleen'), who headed BBC Children's Programmes in

Scotland, and persuaded her to give me an audition. Hoping to make it more interesting and entertaining, I put on a parody of their signature show *Down at the Mains*, but with voices of the characters, farm animal noises and homemade sound effects to try to spice up what I thought was a dull programme.

People stared out in disbelief from the gallery and control room. I don't think they enjoyed the performance much, but they sportingly agreed to put me on a new venture for Children's Hour called *We want to broadcast*. The opportunity, however, never came, and *Down at the Mains* continued in my eyes to be dull as ditchwater. I still felt even as a young lad that there was a missing ingredient to broadcasting in those days.

As I looked back to these early days I wondered what it was that made talks by people like Charles Hill, the 'Radio Doctor', so interesting, even with his lugubrious advice about regular bowels. It was of course his wonderful voice and superb powers of description which kept up the interest. Even our own gym teacher from school, Jack Coleman-Smith, regularly gave an early-morning exercise programme on Scottish radio, with the added interest of his own vocal accompaniment. To the tune of *Waltzing Matilda* he would end his programme by singing, '*If you do your exercises every morning, I'll come a waltzing Matilda with you*'. That was his way of capturing and keeping the listeners' attention on what could have been a dreary programme.

I realised the power of broadcasting as a way of educating people, and watched with particular interest when television made its appearance. Here was a medium which fascinated me, and when my parents bought a twelve-inch Ferguson TV in time for King George VI's funeral in 1952 and later the

Coronation of the Queen, I could hardly contain my excitement.

Returning to my thoughts about improving our training at AMTC, I became more and more convinced that in television we had a medium that could be adapted for use in training our aircrew. I already had the idea of using television cameras for monitoring the wellbeing of the pilot in the decompression chamber, and of course it would be perfect to record our training sessions for teaching purposes. It was an approach that was pretty new then, although of course it has been widely adopted since.

Tom Dobie worked wonders again and somehow managed to secure a very expensive state-of-the-art closed circuit television system for the Centre. There was nothing like it in any other Service training establishment, and I was in my element being able to experiment with this new equipment. It consisted of four cameras, two Phillips tape recorders and numerous monitors of various screen sizes which would be ideal for my purposes. I tried to make some videos, but I didn't have the professional skills to make an educational film or video. Also with the type of recording system of the time it was well-nigh impossible to edit them cleanly.

I wondered how the professionals managed and wanted to find out more, so I went to see a company called ETV (Educational Television) in their studios in Sauchiehall Street in Glasgow. They were piping out programmes to some 300 schools and colleges in the Glasgow area. It was the first closed circuit network to be set up in Europe, and they were a small team of dedicated and highly-skilled people. I was able to watch how it was done and to work out the main techniques and the use of lighting.

I also saw how Scottish Television (STV) were doing it, and managed through Alastair Beaton, Director of the ETV, to get a visit to the Theatre Royal in Glasgow, which Howard and Wyndham Theatre Company, who owned STV at that time, were using as their main studios. I watched the making of *A Song for Scotland* and again learned some tricks of the trade which I knew I could use for my own training purposes.

I even managed an invitation to a TV trade event and exhibition at which I watched the filming of an episode of *Dr Who* with the Daleks, which was all very new at that time. I was concerned at the cramped heat-loading conditions in which poor out-of-work chorus girls operated the Daleks. They were so pleased to have the job that the last thing to concern them was comfort, but I had already mentally designed a cooling system and just wished I could have helped them with that. The same problem would crop up later in my career, and that experience came in very handy.

I was beginning to get somewhere in my quest to look at every available technique that could be used in teaching, and used up most of my leave entitlement for a visit to the United States, where I headed for Hollywood, the home of film and television. The highlight of the holiday break was a visit to Universal Television Studios there. At that time there were no tours of the studios by the public as there are now, but I happened to meet up with a group of film cameramen and technicians in the Brown Derby bar opposite my hotel on Vine Street in Hollywood. Hearing my interest in TV, they invited me to come over to the studio to watch some filming and go behind the scenes to watch the making of some of their earlier productions like *The Torn Curtain* and two television series, one being *McHale's Navy* and the other *The*

Munsters. It was fascinating, and a great privilege to see the tricks of the trade and learn how creative lighting and realistic, detailed modelling could transport you to far-off places when in fact they were being filmed in a studio. This gave me fresh ideas, particularly as the days of huge budget films were almost over and these productions were being made almost on a shoestring. It opened up the possibility that I could do something useful within our Unit's tight budget imposed by the RAF.

Before returning to the UK I visited the Science Museum in Chicago and was fascinated to see youngsters and adults alike crawling over and into a giant model of the human heart. Immediately I saw the potential for aircrew training, and I resolved to acquire some medical models which would help in our teaching of human body systems – just as one of my test pilot colleagues hoped might happen one day.

Back at North Luffenham, using the information I had gained, I set up quite a professional little studio with curtains borrowed from the NAAFI and two cameras. Studio lighting was provided by aircraft hangar lights, which kept blowing the circuit breakers and at times plunging the Centre into darkness.

I started making training videos, which were very successful, and I was now in my element because I was combining my two passions, aviation physiology and broadcasting. I gave interviews for ATV in the Midlands and some of the other local and national television companies, who were now clamouring to see and film the work of the Centre. I was now well on my way to climbing one of the other branches of the 'tree of life' which Mr McCabe had urged me to draw. Indeed, life and work at North Luffenham and the Centre were going well, and the morale of the team led by Tom Dobie was at an all-time high. We were all proud of the huge progress we had made at AMTC. I was in my element, and felt that my hard work had been very worthwhile.

Then in April 1965 came the devastating news that the Government had cancelled the TSR2 aircraft. It had just completed its test flights and promised to be the all-singing and all-dancing aircraft that we were looking forward to. It went faster and further and carried a bigger missile payload than its predecessors. Everything we were doing to build up the training programme was in anticipation of this aeroplane coming into production, so the announcement was the worst possible news.

There was astonishment and then deep disappointment in the aircraft industry. There was gloom in the Services, with the realisation that all their hard work had been in vain. Morale sank to a new low when newspapers carried pictures of the wonderful new aeroplane being unceremoniously broken up in some MoD scrapyard.

Like the rest of the staff of AMTC, I sank to the bottom of my cage. Like them I feared for the future, and couldn't get over the thought that all our work building up the Centre to meet the needs of the TSR2 and other new aircraft had been slashed in one blow. I decided that I must visit John Ernsting at the IAM to help me sort out what my next move ought to be.

'I know exactly how you feel' he said. 'We are all devastated at IAM by this rotten blow. We've had to cancel major experiments and change projects because of it. To be honest Gordon, none of us here knows what's going to happen next.'

He listened sympathetically as I explained my devastation that all our changes at AMTC would finish up on the scrapheap too.

'Not at all' said John. 'I have always worked on the principle that when one door closes another opens. It's what we make of any situation that counts. We need to go through that door and look for new opportunities and new directions. The days of lengthy expensive research projects at IAM are now over. We're going to have to adapt to different requirements in aviation medicine and physiology. We're going to have to look for crucial experiments that will give us answers quickly. It doesn't mean dropping standards, just that we must now use our resources and equipment more efficiently.'

I was greatly encouraged by John's wisdom, which reminded me of a saying I had once heard: 'It's not the strongest but the most adaptive that survive'. I could almost see the cogwheels spinning in John's fertile mind, and instantly knew he was hatching another plan. I didn't know at the time what it might be, and I had absolutely no inkling that it would open a new door in my own life and career.

The first clue as to what John was thinking came when he asked me to join him and a member of the Human Engineering Department of RAE in a visit to the USAF base at Alconbury. This was strange. JE and most of the lab had little or no communication with the Human Engineers and relationships with them were distinctly frosty, even although they were just across the runway from IAM. What was up, I wondered?

We met up in the Officers' Club at USAF Alconbury. The Base Commander took us round the base, showing us all the facilities and pointing out the various aircraft operating from there. Out of the blue, JE asked if there was any chance that he might have a look into the cockpit of a Phantom. Now, the cockpit of that aircraft held a vast array of highly secret weaponry and sophisticated electronics which were a closely guarded secret. I was certain the request would be turned down flat.

'Sure thing, I can try' said the General. 'Why don't you have me talk to the guys in Washington?' So saying, he picked up a telephone handset and from the car asked to be patched in to the Pentagon in Washington. This was long before there were mobile phones and easy international communication, and for me it was particularly amazing that he could contact the States from a moving staff car. I was agog and listened in wonderment as he spoke to someone at the other end of the phone across the Atlantic.

Finally he came off the phone. 'OK guys, I believe the game's on' he said. I turned and looked at JE. 'Is this the other door opening?' I whispered. He smiled and said 'Hmm, possibly, just let's see'.

We drove up to a slightly sinister-looking USAF Phantom sitting outside a hangar and with one leap, JE bounded up the steps. He peered for ages into the cockpit. Then I knew that one of the replacements for the ill-fated TSR2 was going be the American F4 Phantom. How exciting, I thought, good old JE. I instantly felt much more optimistic for the future.

It was a few weeks after that visit to Alconbury that John phoned and asked me if I would like to consider coming back to Institute of Aviation Medicine. He explained that they were joining forces with the human engineering people at RAE Farnborough to examine the requirements for the new US F4 Phantom II. It confirmed my guess that it would be coming in to service with the RAF as a replacement for the TSR2.

The protective equipment and assemblies used in the USAF version of the aircraft were quite different from ours, and John explained that there would need to be a complete revamp and redesign of them for use in the RAF version. He was in the process of setting up a team to look at every aspect of that conversion process and said he wanted me to lead the project on his behalf.

I couldn't believe my ears. This was the breakthrough I had longed for. It was the other door opening up, and it brought new horizons and the chance to prove my worth to the RAF Medical Branch and the Institute. It was just the work I had wanted to be involved in for so long; I would be at the sharp end of military air operations and I couldn't say yes fast enough. The future was beginning to look just a little bit brighter again.

CHAPTER SEVEN

SPREADING MY WINGS

I will never forget my excitement on taking up my new posting back at the Institute of Aviation Medicine at Farnborough. This was what I had dreamed about from the start of my Service career, and now I was going there as project team leader for what became known as the Phantom Fitting Trial. It was a major departure from the usual work of the Institute and in setting it up John Ernsting had put into practice what he preached. He had adapted to modern requirements and had managed to bring together scientists and experts from the RAE Human Engineering Department, something which had previously been thought an impossibility, as well as involving doctors, scientists and technicians from every Section and Division of the lab. The project would involve a mix of expertise ranging from test pilots and doctors to ex-army tailors, technicians, MoD representatives and so on. It was a remarkable achievement by John; in fact it was history in the making.

The first phase of the fitting trial went on for more than a year. John had arranged for the RAE technical people to build a wooden mock-up of the Phantom, a perfect replica complete with all the switches, controls and instruments to the exact dimensions of the aeroplane. Aircrew wearing the full test assemblies were assessed for their ability to reach switches and operate controls, so we knew that by the end of the trial we would have a perfect match of the man to the machine he was flying.

Over the trial period I worked harder than I had ever worked before. I was eating and sleeping aviation medicine and physiology, but I didn't mind a bit. John was working on the design of new miniature oxygen regulators that would meet the operational requirements of new aircraft coming into service with the RAF. Between times I would join him in his work and squeeze into my own busy schedule the altitude trials of the oxygen equipment in the decompression chambers. With the frantic demands on the Division, I often had to represent him at meetings with manufacturers and the MoD. Life seemed to be a whirlwind of work and experimentation. I was back in my element again.

As the trial progressed, we moved into the second phase of adapting to new requirements. More developments appeared, which again were departures from the normal pattern of work at IAM. A new Section was built up called the Aircrew Equipment Group (AEG), responsible for testing every new aircraft-specific assembly coming into service with the RAF and Royal Navy. Assessments in the cockpit mock-ups were followed by real operational flight trials undertaken by the two pilots who were permanently attached to the Division, using a Canberra bomber and a Hunter T4 training aircraft.

I tried to participate in as many in-flight trials as I could, although at times they realistically exposed quite a few minor but practical issues. During one test flight one of our IAM pilots had flown out over the sea, and as soon as he was all dressed up and airborne he found he needed a pee. That was fine, because they were about to test a 'piddle pack' which jellified the urine, but he then realised that he had put his long johns on the wrong way round! His co-pilot suggested using a dinghy knife to free his 'equipment', but he retorted 'There's no way you're coming anywhere near my family jewels with that thing!' After that occurrence I took even more care in donning my flying clothing assemblies before flying.

As John Ernsting had promised, the final phase of the project involved familiarising operational aircrew with the work we were doing at IAM. This, to my delight, took us out to the real 'sharp end' of military flying - the operational RAF Stations. We visited countless front line flying stations to demonstrate the new equipment to the aircrew.

On one of these visits I had an interesting experience. We flew out from Farnborough in the Canberra bomber to RAF Gutersloh in Germany, and were put up overnight in the Officers' Mess there. It had been a Luftwaffe Mess during World War 2 and it clearly hadn't changed very much since those days. Downstairs was the bar where the German fliers used to congregate and no doubt boast about their 'kills' over a stein of beer.

Upstairs in the tower of the Mess was a room known as Göring's Room. Legend has it that Reichsmarschall Göring, head of the Luftwaffe, used this part of the Mess to boast about his own wartime exploits, probably exaggerating and almost certainly boring the new generation of pilots out of their minds. The room was still furnished very much as it had been in Göring's day. There was the original solid oak table surrounded by matching oak chairs bearing the sign of the swastika carved into the back of each seat.

It is said that one of Göring's favourite expressions was 'If I should tell a lie may the beam above my head crack'. Apparently, one of the young German pilots arranged for the beam above Göring's head to be sawn through so that by a system of chains, pulleys and a hidden lever it would appear to crack and drop from the ceiling, finishing up just above the Reichsmarschall's head whenever he spoke his favourite phrase. The system still worked, and I was allowed to sit at the top of the table and witness the same trick with the beam that Göring had experienced many years before.

This new approach by the Altitude and other Divisions of the Institute helped to spread the word about all the aviation medical research coming out of Farnborough, and we attempted to dispel the myth that we all lived in 'ivory towers'. But one unwelcome situation developed in 1967 which opened the whole of the Royal Aircraft Establishment to a measure of ridicule. It started with newspaper headlines that proclaimed there had been an 'INVASION BY ALIENS'. For days the No 1 Mess at Farnborough buzzed with the news that the police and RAF had been flooded with telephone calls from the public reporting the discovery of six small 'flying saucers' in locations in a perfect line across southern England from Sheppey to the Bristol Channel. It turned out to be a 'War of the Worlds' rag week stunt carried out by engineering apprentices from the RAE and students from the nearby Farnborough Technical College. All hell broke loose in the Farnborough and Aldershot areas, which became overrun with police, army and bomb disposal experts. They found that the 'flying saucers' were filled with a foul-smelling brown liquid that stank of sewage. It was in fact just that - human excrement! The game was up when they discovered some Exide batteries among the contents of the supposedly alien saucers.

Everything calmed down eventually, but the fact that the hoax had originated from the 'boffin-land' of Farnborough brought forth many crude jokes from aircrew (including some at our expense) – most of them referring to the brown, evil-smelling liquid content found in the hoax flying saucers!

Despite this minor setback the IAM and all its various Divisions continued to grow in stature. In the Altitude Division we plodded on with our work designing and testing new oxygen systems, and became heavily involved with miniature versions which could be mounted on an oxygen mask or on the chest of the aviator. Thanks to John Ernsting I was working in close collaboration with the RAE engineers and absorbing many of their engineering skills. When I eventually put together all the work I had done as a thesis, I submitted it to Glasgow University, Department of Physiology in candidature for a PhD. It apparently was the first submission in the field of aviation physiology, and I was awarded the doctorate in 1970.

So novel was the combination of physiology and engineering that I was invited to submit my thesis to the Royal Aeronautical Society for the award of a Certificate of Engineering. However I declined to do so, although I gratefully accepted Membership of the Society instead. I couldn't help thinking how proud my old Dad would have been. It was a combination of medicine, science and engineering of which he would most certainly have approved.

My happiness soared to new heights when a new light came into my life – a lovely girl who from almost the first meeting simply bowled me over. Her name was Christina (Kirstie) Livingstone, and her parents had just retired to the town of Fortrose, near to where my elderly mother lived. I first met her at a party when I was on leave and couldn't keep my eyes off her. I had never really believed in love at first sight, but somehow I knew immediately that she would be someone very, very special in my life.

I played it quite cool until I saw the lie of the land. I was so scared that with the distance between Farnborough and Fortrose I might lose her in the same way I had lost Heather.

I needn't have been too worried, as reports came through by way of my mother that Kirstie had feelings towards me too. As time went on I took every opportunity I could get to go up north and even drove up overnight to spend the odd weekend at home, on the off chance that we might meet up.

When the MoD asked me to look at a problem of carbon monoxide poisoning in winch operators of RAF Target Towing Launches, they assumed I would plump immediately for the work, as it was being carried out in RAF Luqa in Malta. They simply couldn't understand why I chose the almost unknown Marine Craft Unit at RAF Alness in the north of Scotland to carry out the investigation. The reason was that it was only about half an hour away from Fortrose, and it would give me the opportunity to see more of Kirstie.

My colleagues at IAM too thought that I must be completely mad to turn down the opportunity to visit sunny

Malta. I heard later that because of my choice the lab had been complimented by MoD on the speed of response to their request and praised for choosing the least expensive option. Only John Ernsting and a few close colleagues and friends knew the real reason for my unusual choice.

I don't know whether it was that work that earned me for a short time the nickname of 'Speedy Sharp', but I was curious to know how that had started. John Ernsting was known as 'Commander Energy' for obvious reasons, and David Denison, who worked in the Division, was called 'Denison of the Deep', on account of his great interest in and experience of diving and underwater physiology. As for my own nickname it seemed to reflect the recognition by the MoD that no-matter how unusual or complicated the project, our Division could be relied upon to tackle it swiftly and carry it out accurately and without fuss. Perhaps because of this reputation we began to get more and more of this type of request from MoD Departments, as well as other organisations. We took on an unusual and very wide variety of aeromedical and physiological projects and were constantly being asked for permission to use our chambers and other research facilities. With my new reputation it was often old 'Speedy' who would be roped in to help them out. However bizarre the request, I was always eager to oblige and participate, knowing that I was building up experience in field research techniques that would be useful in the future.

In 1966 an approach came from the organisers of the Daily Mirror World Cup Rally, which was going from London to Mexico and passing through La Paz in Bolivia, more than 11,000 feet above sea level. It was in La Paz during a pre-rally inspection of the route that one of the cars had a puncture, and when the crew got out to fix it they collapsed from hypoxia because of the altitude. Paddy Hopkirk, who finished fourth in the rally (which was won by a country mile by Hannu Mikkola in a Ford Escort), was sceptical about the need for oxygen, so we put him in the decompression chamber, took him up to 11,500 feet and showed him the effects of lack of oxygen. When we brought the chamber back down to ground level and showed Paddy his feeble efforts to make even the simplest calculations at altitude, he completely appreciated the devastating effects of lack of oxygen on skilled rally driving. After that experience he was only too pleased to use the oxygen system that the Division put together, and he used it during the actual rally.

HRH Prince Michael of Kent also came along – he took part in the rally but in the event failed to finish. He too was keen to experience the effects of altitude on the drivers, so we put him through the same hypoxia experience that Paddy had undergone. That convinced him of the need for all drivers to carry oxygen in the Rally.

My own interest in cars continued, although I had replaced the Ferrari with a much more docile Triumph GT6. It was called the 'poor man's E-Type Jaguar' and I got great use and a lot of fun out of that car without the crippling expense of maintenance I had had with the Ferrari. Just as well, because I now began to turn my attention to a very different type of transport and one that I became totally absorbed in – flying.

During my time in the Middle East I had been able to get my hands on a huge variety of aircraft, and to a large extent had satisfied my longing to fly. However I now felt that it was time to extend my knowledge and skills of flying, take formal flying lessons and get my private licence. My old friend Don Cameron, now at Farnborough, was an instructor, and I took lessons from him sometimes in the Tiger Moth biplane he flew from Leicester East airfield. On other occasions he gave me formal instruction in Cherokees belonging to the Three Counties Aero Club at Blackbushe Aerodrome. He was a brilliant instructor and I couldn't have found a better. During my time at AMTC I noticed how Don could relate well to visiting aircrew and hoped that some of his skills would rub off on me.

I took to flying in a big way, although I had a bit of adventure when it was time to take the long-distance solo flight. That involved following a triangular route between Blackbushe, Oxford, Sandown (Isle of Wight) and back to Blackbushe. I was really enjoying the flight, but stupidly made a classic error; in setting off on one of the legs of the journey, I forgot to reset my direction indicator. The direction indicator is based on a gyroscope, and if you don't orientate it when you start, it doesn't know where it is, and neither do you. I was soon lost and very worried indeed. I was looking out for the runway at Thruxton racetrack, but I couldn't spot it to save my life. Nothing matched between ground and map, and the anxiety level was beginning to rise.

At last I recognised the long runway at Boscombe Down, called them up and got permission to land. They thought I was a VIP who was due to pay them a visit that day, so there was some embarrassment and confusion when they found out the truth. I took off again, having taken particular care to reset the direction indicator gyro, and returned to Blackbushe, arriving just within my allotted time.

It could have been worse. One cadet had made the same

mistake and set out for the Isle of Wight. He thought Southampton Water seemed rather wider than he'd expected, and all was revealed when he finally finished up in a Dutch tulip field and realised that he had crossed the Channel. At least I was not alone in making this error, but I learned never to repeat it again.

It was during the learning phase, that I had a strange and somewhat unnerving encounter as I was returning on a solo flight to Blackbushe. The voice of Pete Hooper in Blackbushe control tower warned me to be on the lookout for a Shackleton bomber coming in on my port bow at low level. A strange piece of information, I thought, but I looked around; I couldn't spot it. As I looked down from the aeroplane I saw that in the grounds of the imposing Minley Manor there were sentry boxes and fluttering swastika banners. I could even make out soldiers wearing Nazi uniforms, and on the path leading up to the Manor House were a German military halftrack vehicle and a motorcycle and sidecar.

I was utterly confused and wondered if toxic fumes had entered the cockpit, causing me to hallucinate. If I had been flying in the deserts of the Middle East I might have put it down to a mirage effect, but at the time there was no rational explanation for the phenomenon. It wasn't until I visited a pub near Blackbushe called the Crown and Cushion (or to give it its nickname, because it was always busy, the 'Crowd and Push In'). The barman there explained that a film company was shooting a film called *Mosquito Squadron* over at Minley Manor because it bore a marked resemblance to Amiens Jail in France. From cameras fitted to the nose of the Shackleton I had been warned to look out for, they were filming the scene of a successful low level pinpoint bombing raid on the jail by the RAF during WW2. This remarkable achievement helped to release captured SO (Special Operations) prisoners.

The filming had reportedly gone very well, but the rather miserable-looking man standing next to me at the bar (in charge of special effects, it turned out) told me his patience was just about exhausted - as soon as he built up his set, including laying brick walls, the film director blew it up again. He had to endure retake after retake, and he was not a happy bunny. He managed to raise a smile when I told him of my strange experience flying over the film set. For my part, I was greatly relieved at the confirmation that I had not been suffering from a toxic illusional state during my flight.

Having finally passed all the exams and flights required, I got my Private Pilot's Licence and joined the RAE flying club, which meant I got to fly the light aircraft that were kept there in the club hangar. I toyed with the notion of buying a Wallis gyrocopter and had discussed the possibility when Ken Wallis the designer had visited the Institute. It was very new and the gyrocopter had just come into production, but I was not sure whether I had the skills to fly such an unconventional aeroplane. I gave up the idea.

I did not regret it. A year later, as Duty Medical Officer at the Farnborough Air show, I watched a display gyrocopter go out of control during a tight turn manoeuvre and crash to the ground before my eyes. By the time I got to the wreckage the very experienced display pilot was unfortunately dead. I was saddened by that. I was not put off the idea of eventually owning my own aircraft, although I decided to stick to a fixed-wing model if was ever able to attain such a dream.

That was when my mother stepped in and very kindly offered to help me to buy a conventional aeroplane. I had seen the one I longed for advertised in *Aeroplane* magazine. It was a little two-seater Piper Colt with a tricycle undercarriage, built for the US market. Its registration letters were G-ARJG and I immediately nicknamed it 'Julie Golf' after the letters 'JG' in the registration. I loved that little aeroplane, and flying it was like driving a car. I bought it from the West London Flying Club at White Waltham and installed it in a small blister hangar just below IAM that gave easy access to the main runway.

Don and I flew many times in Julie Golf. We tried to fly north to Inverness Dalcross Airport so that I could show my mother what her stake in the world of light aviation looked like, but the weather clamped down and we had to land at Newcastle. We stayed in the St George's Hotel, which had been an old RAF Officers' Mess I used to visit at Middleton St George. It felt strange to see the place full of civilians with not a uniform in sight, but the break was a welcome one and I was glad we hadn't pressed on in such bad weather. Don was much too experienced and wise for that to happen.

Mother had to wait a while longer before she could see the Piper Colt. She announced she was coming down to Farnborough and wanted to fly in the aeroplane. What I knew she really meant was that she wanted to have a shot at the controls, as flying was something she had never accomplished in her early active years.

She was a natural and enjoyed the flight. For some reason I didn't quite understand at the time she asked me never to take Kirstie up in the Colt. I don't think this was any reflection on my own flying abilities, more a case of being prematurely protective perhaps, about the person she saw as a future daughter-in-law. Even when the opportunity later presented itself, I stuck to my word and Kirstie, much to her disappointment, never got to fly in 'Julie Golf'.

Later Don and I managed to fly the Piper Colt over the English Channel, but before take-off from Farnborough we witnessed the sad sight of the RAE club glider making a nosedive into the main runway. It crashed in a cloud of dust and debris. We stopped and leaped out the aeroplane, but we were too late to save the poor glider pilot, who was already dead. It was a chap I had met a few times, and that experience took the edge off the subsequent flight across the Channel.

After making the crossing we flew up and down the Normandy beaches, stopping off at Ostend Airport. After the return flight across the Channel we landed back at Manston Airfield for Customs clearance. I was taken aback when the young customs officer asked if I had a bar aboard the aircraft. This was a technical term which I didn't know at the time, and I jokingly replied that we had a cocktail bar at the front and a public bar at the rear. This remark was met with a frosty look, but the customs officer was not officious and after Don explained that I was still under training and not familiar with procedures he let us go on our way back to Farnborough. Don gave me a stern warning never to joke with HM Customs, as it could run the risk of the aeroplane being stripped down to bare bones in their search for smuggled items.

My love of flying grew stronger. I was in the enviable position of being able as part of my work to fly in the Institute's aircraft by day and in my own little Piper Colt in the Summer evenings and at weekends. Little did I think that the two flying activities would merge and that a chance observation in my recreational flying would lead to a new and even more exciting phase in my career.

One day when I was flying in the Colt back to Farnborough, I spotted a huge anvil-shaped cloud in the distance. I knew this meant bad weather, so I made an attempt to get into calmer air above the thunderclouds. I started to climb to higher altitude, but the heating system couldn't cope with carburettor de-icing and the engine revs started to drop in a most worrying way. There was nothing for it but to attempt to fly round the blackening clouds, and if necessary turn back and divert to another airfield.

The weather was worsening, and perhaps stupidly I decided to press on, but I ran into very nasty turbulence – the worst I had ever experienced. The little aeroplane began to buffet in a most alarming manner and I was thankful for my seatbelt to stop me from being flung around the cockpit. The whole aeroplane vibrated like mad, and I found it difficult to maintain straight and level flight. Visibility was terrible and I had to go on to instrument flying.

I was reminded of the stories my father used to tell me about Alcock and Brown making the first transatlantic crossing. They met similar bad weather situations to those I was now facing, yet with a calm approach and skilful flying they managed to survive the ordeal. Although I was terrified out of my wits, I followed their example, and by a stroke of luck I managed to clear the filthy weather, find clear air and return to more pleasant flying. I landed safe and sound, glad to be back in the safety of Farnborough.

I recalled that during that difficult flight I had noticed that throughout the bad spell of turbulence the rate and depth of my breathing had increased and I had begun to get some tingling in my lips and a feeling of light-headedness. These I knew to be the symptoms and signs of hyperventilation or overbreathing, like the well-known playground trick where if you deliberately breathe quickly and deeply you can get muzzy-headed and pass out in a faint. It might have been fun in the playground, but it wasn't so funny when it came to flying.

I wondered what had caused this condition. Fear and anxiety were known to bring it on, and I had certainly had a good deal of that. There had never to my knowledge been any suggestion that the intense concentration of instrument flying could cause it - but if it had, then I realised I might have made a new discovery. The most likely cause seemed to me to be the intense whole-body vibration brought about by the buffeting in the aeroplane. I was determined to explore this potential flying hazard and discussed my observations with my colleagues at IAM.

John Ernsting was interested to hear about my experience. The Institute had been asked to look into incident reports filed by RAF pilots. Some had noticed feelings of light-headedness and slight detachment when flying at high speed and low level over mountains and through valleys in terrain-hugging exercise flights. All reported turbulence in the low-altitude thicker air. I was amused to think that my experiences in the little Piper Colt were being compared to those of the finest and most highly-trained pilots in the RAF, flying the most sophisticated aeroplanes of the day.

John had done some early work on whole body vibration and its effects on breathing, and he asked me to follow this up with a new project which would involve flying in the Institute's Hunter and Canberra aircraft and carrying out a full-scale laboratory study. I was over the Moon at what had to be the best project ever offered to me. I felt that my passion for flying was now being fulfilled, and I set about this new challenge with great gusto.

A new whole-body vibrator facility had recently been installed at the Institute, but I wasn't able to use it for my research project because it was out of commission while experts examined its forty-foot shaft and carried out the necessary safety checks. In any case it was capital equipment belonging to another Division and they had first priority when it came back on line.

I turned to the possibility of modifying an earlier experimental version - a simple vibrating platform model. The technical staff practically rebuilt the old model and fixed a disarmed aircraft ejection seat on to the vibrating platform. Preliminary trials confirmed that at certain frequencies the experimental subjects suffered marked discomfort as the body's organs went into sympathetic resonance. This in turn frequently led to hyperventilation and diminution of consciousness, just like the episode I experienced in the Colt and suspiciously similar to the incidents reported by RAF pilots. Could vibration be one of possibly several causes of the condition in high speed low-level flying?

There was only one way to find out. We really had to mount a full-scale investigation. I was given a small team for the laboratory part of the project. With the requirement to test miniature oxygen systems in flight as part of my other work, I was able to fly in all kinds of conditions and extend the vibration studies to real situations.

One of the phrases everyone at the lab dreaded was, "If you're not doing anything, do you fancy going for a spin?"

Accepting this invitation could mean spending half the day whirling around in the centrifuge with needles in every available blood vessel, never a pleasant experience!

But as was the custom at IAM, everybody participated in each other's projects and experiments. A ride on the vibrator was pretty unpleasant at times, and we had some difficulty finding volunteers – until one day I came back from lunch to find a queue of people all wanting to have a go. Word had got out that at a certain frequency the prostate gland went into sympathetic resonance and people claimed that they were getting ten-minute orgasms! Of course it was just a rumour someone had put about for mischief, but I did nothing to dispel that myth until the experiment was over.

With the benefit of a larger than usual number of experimental subjects we got excellent and reproducible results. The outcome of this project certainly raised my standing in the IAM, and I hope made a useful contribution to flying safety -which after all, is what it is all about.

I was rather disappointed that a more extensive study into hyperventilation in flight was not possible at the time. John Ernsting, however, came up with a brilliant interim solution. Why not let us adopt the NASA approach to some of the hazards in spaceflight? If they cannot easily and quickly overcome a problem, they build it into their training programme as part of astronaut familiarisation. We could do the same, and include it as part of our training at AMTC.

This was excellent. It was something we could implement straight away at no cost to MoD and the Institute. 'One day' John sighed, 'we might be able to look in depth at the problem and tackle it in the more traditional IAM ways.'

Many years later Dr Mike Gibson, a former colleague of

mine at IAM, did just that. He made an in-depth study of hyperventilation in flight and wrote a paper reviewing the condition. He confirmed the difficulties he had encountered in measuring its effects on pilots in flight and emphasised the importance of training aircrew to recognise early symptoms of the condition.

As it turned out, John Ernsting's stopgap solution may have proved to be effective. The reported incidence of the condition in flight seemed to decline from then on.

The orgasm rumour was always a source of amusement to audiences when I gave lectures and presented papers to scientific and medical bodies. But what made matters worse was that when I used several clips of high-speed cine film to illustrate my presentations, they clearly showed both my nipples rotating in response to one of the vibration frequencies. This led to the suggestion from colleagues and aircrew that I ought to stick a tassel on each nipple and audition for a variety act in a Soho joint. They assured me I could make a fortune. Needless to say that was one change in my career path that I didn't wish to explore!

Later, when I wrote up the results of this work on vibration and hyperventilation, I submitted it as a thesis to Glasgow University for consideration of the award of MD (Doctorate of Medicine). It was I believe the first thesis they had received for work in the field of aerospace medicine and I was awarded the degree with commendation. I was so glad that my mother was able to be present at the graduation ceremony at Glasgow University, knowing that her help in purchasing the Piper Colt had played a tiny but significant role in sparking off my research work into flight safety. She was pleased as Punch at the notion.

'With a bit of luck you might get to fly in Concorde' said John Ernsting one day. 'The lab is going to get involved again in aviation medical problems when they come to test fly the aeroplane.'

I pricked up my ears - flying experience just couldn't get better than that. Concorde had been on the drawing board for some time, and on 11 December 1967 the first prototype was unveiled at the Aerospatiale plant in Toulouse in southern France. The aeroplane would be going up to 60,000 feet, higher than any previous passenger aircraft. John Ernsting had previously advised on the risks of loss of cabin pressure at such a high altitude and had suggested as a safety precaution that the windows should be small and oval in shape to reduce the risk of cracking through fatigue and causing an explosive decompression. He had calculated that even if two of the smaller windows blew out at the same moment there would be enough time for the pilots to bring the aeroplane down to safer heights.

Later we were asked to assist the two British test pilots, John Cochrane and Brian Trubshaw, who were going to be doing the first high-altitude test flights. We kitted them up with an oxygen system and a partial pressure suit with a helmet. An Anglo-French Aeromedical Committee was set up and I went to all the meetings as the IAM representative. They were held in the control tower at Heathrow, in Paris or Toulouse in France.

Unfortunately the French, including their pilot, André Turcat, proved very difficult to work with. We saw Gallic arrogance at its worst; everything had to be translated into French line by line, although they all spoke perfectly good English. Matters came to a head when the French team demonstrated an oxygen system designed to keep crew conscious in the event of a loss of cabin pressure. It was an excellent system and was soon adopted. They had prepared a mock-up of Concorde's flight deck which was dimensionally correct, and had fitted the proposed oxygen system to a panel at the side ready to go. But John Cochrane was not in a good mood, and he took an instant dislike to the French boffin. He took his cup of coffee and simply emptied it straight on to the box that housed the system, flooding it with hot coffee and ruined it. He wanted to make the point that the lid of the container offered the crew the perfect place for putting a cup of coffee.

The French team went apoplectic, but he had a point, and the device was eventually produced with an apex so that it could not be used as a miniature coffee table, but it was perhaps hardly the most diplomatic way to make it. Unfortunately it was John Cochrane's well-known style.

The aeromedical aspects of Concorde took me somewhat away from the intensity of military aviation and brought me into the civilian world for a while. It was a refreshing and enjoyable chapter in my life, and I loved it. I never managed to get my flight during the test phase of Concorde, although it was a marvellous sight to behold when it made its debut flight at the Farnborough Air Show and later went into service with British Airways.

My days of intense flying at the Institute were now beginning to ebb a little bit and the last in-flight study I was asked to carry out for the RAF was in 1969. It proved to be rather an interesting experience and not quite what I would have expected as my 'swan song'. It was called the 'VC 10 Frozen

Food Concept' – an attempt to introduce frozen meals into troop-carrying aircraft on long haul flights. There was a worry that the dry ice which kept the food cold for the duration of the flight might release carbon dioxide gas which would drift into the flight deck and compromise the safety of the aircrew.

I joined forces with a scientist from ICI Agricultural Division who was an expert in the field of frozen food. Together we devised a measuring device which would monitor the escape of CO_2 gas in flight. The only way we could set up our equipment was to thread a tube through a hole in the forward lavatory with the sensor reaching down into the forward freight hold where the food containers were stored.

Yes, you've guessed it - it meant that I had to spend much of the flight in the lavatory, taking regular readings. Fortunately there were compensations. First, we stopped off for a few days at each RAF Station in Cyprus, Bahrain, Gan in the Maldives and finally Changi in Singapore and in each port of call the catering team demonstrated the new in-flight meals while the aircrew, the ICI boffin and I were free to take a mini holiday - or so we thought. The other compensation was that we were encouraged to consume as many steaks and other in-flight goodies as we could eat. After a while the novelty wore off and I couldn't face another steak meal for the duration of the trip.

I had a great time in RAF Akrotiri in Cyprus, although it was spoiled somewhat when a feral cat in a café beat me to a kebab and plunged its teeth into my hand in the process. I worried for the rest of the trip that I might get rabies and die a horrible death, but all was well until on the next stopover on the journey in Gan, where I stupidly fell asleep under a coconut palm tree and suffered a dreadful dose of sunburn of the face.

When we reached Singapore the Medical Officer responsible for hygiene on the station took me to an outdoor eatery. Rats were running up and down the storm ditch, and although he assured me that the red hot wok would kill off any germs from my food I was still a little anxious about the outcome if he was wrong. I survived that one, but I had an unpleasant experience at a barbecue held on a sand spit in Changi Creek opposite the Officers' Mess. It was not the food this time that caused the problem but a drunken army officer who offered to paddle me back to the Mess in his two-man canoe. He dropped me off on the muddy shore just short of the dry land of the Mess garden, and I had an awful struggle to avoid being sucked down into the mud with every step I took. With a frantic effort and mustering my last drop of energy I just managed to reach the safety of dry land, caked in foul-smelling mud but thankful to have survived another unexpected experience.

With the results we got from the project we managed to reassure the aircrew that they would not be affected by the frozen meals carried aboard their aircraft. Everyone was happy at the outcome, and that, strangely enough, included me. I had yet again gained so much from the study, despite the unpredicted dangers of the investigation.

My flying experiences over the past years had marked an advance up a branch of the tree of life that Mr McCabe had urged me to draw as schoolboy. My passion and craving for flying had now been fully satiated. The opportunity to add yet another equally exciting branch was to come in quite an unexpected way, marking another turning point in my work and my life.

CHAPTER EIGHT

ON AIR, AND DOWN TO EARTH

One day 'Roxy' Roxburgh (who was now Commandant of IAM following the death of Bill Stewart) approached me out of the blue and asked me how I would feel about getting involved in the Space Rescue Working Group. That word 'space' was one I had been longing to hear ever since Sputnik, and I felt that at last this might be my chance. I had been trying everything I could think of to get into space medicine and had deeply regretted not being involved when Apollo 11 triumphed by putting the first men on the Moon in July 1969.

Roxy said he had taken the working group on, but was finding it too much with all the meetings and conferences it entailed. He knew I was desperate to work in space, as it were; I never knew whether he was passing this on to me because he really couldn't find the time or just to give me a slice of the cake, but if so it was a kind gesture.

The 'space race' was now well under way. During the 1960s we'd had Project Mercury, which put the first

American astronauts in space, and its successor, Project Gemini, the forerunner to the Apollo Moon missions. With all these missions there was an increasing likelihood that at some point there would be a crisis in space and a rescue mission would have to be mounted.

At last the IAM was beginning to appreciate the value of its work to the space programme. John Ernsting had advised on the danger of an oxygen-rich mixture in the cabin of the spacecraft at launch. Such a mixture had led to the drastic and tragic fire on Apollo 1, and John advised that a low-oxygen launch gas mixture in the spacecraft cabin would give much less fire risk and could later be topped up to the required breathing mixture after the craft cleared the launch pad.

John and I discussed the possibilities of an in-flight accident or incident, including the ability of the life-support systems to prevent severe hypoxia. This involved looking at the extreme limits of survival for a crew in difficulties in space. I was particularly interested in finding out how feasible a rescue might be at different stages of a mission.

I even ventured to ask for the use of a computer to help in the complex calculations involved – almost unheard of in the early 1970s. The Institute managed to acquire an analogue computer, and I was authorised to go on a one-week computing course at Burgess Hill near Brighton. I used my new skill to look at every trajectory of a rocket between Earth and Moon and developed a list of possible trajectories for the manned spacecraft. It was clear that a rescue would have to involve another spacecraft sitting ready with a crew of fully-trained astronauts. That simply was not practical, and NASA knew it. Werner von Braun, who had designed the rocket that would take men to the Moon, had put paid to that idea for purely practical reasons. Instead, their policy was to make sure nothing went wrong in the first place - a gamble, as of course it is impossible to be sure. But the question was – if something did go wrong, would there be any chance of someone on the ground intervening?

No one had seriously dared to ask that question in 1970, but all that would soon change. I kept the plots of all the trajectories I had worked out and it wasn't long before I would have reason to be glad of them. Although Apollo 12, our second Moon landing in November 1969, attracted far less media attention than its predecessor, it was actually a very successful and interesting mission. The astronauts spent far longer on the surface of the Moon than they had with Apollo 11 – nearly eight hours compared with two and a half – and embarked on some proper exploring.

There had been a steady increase in the informal exchange of information between the Institute and NASA. We frequently flew across the Atlantic to attend meetings and the Americans were very open about what NASA was doing. They had their own aviation medical experts, although the flight surgeons who were in attendance were more focused on the general health of the astronauts than on how the human body copes in space.

I was particularly impressed by the work of the physiologists at the USAF School of Aviation Medicine (SAM) in San Antonio, and at NASA itself. Our co-operation with the Americans started with a professional exchange of information, each wanting to learn from the other. These visits helped the two-way flow of knowledge and expertise, because we were all fellow professionals talking to each other. Our common aim was to get man safely to the Moon, work there and return safely to Earth.

My opportunity to broadcast on national TV came with the first Apollo mission to go wrong, the ill-fated Apollo 13 in April 1970. The TV channels, who were getting bored with the space race, had more or less ignored Apollo 12 and were about to ignore Apollo 13 as well, until news came on April 13 (that unlucky number again) that with the mission some 50,000 miles out from the Moon there had been an explosion on board. Suddenly all eyes were on TV sets as the world waited for news of the fate of the three astronauts, Jim Lovell, Jack Swigert and Fred Haise.

Roxy had received the news earlier that morning and asked me to represent IAM as their expert on in-flight incidents and space matters. I was flattered to be chosen, as it was something I had been desperately trying to get involved in for years.

He asked me to go to the ITN studios in London, initially to brief Peter Fairley, the Science Editor, on the feasibility of mounting a rescue in space. On arrival I was shown into the Green Room, which was packed with people as it was budget day. Everyone was knocking back gin and tonics and tucking into smoked salmon sandwiches. I got chatting to one chap, and it seemed he had spotted the slide rule sticking out of my briefcase.

I was taken aback when he asked me what I thought we might expect in the Budget from the Chancellor. I breezily responded 'I expect he'll give us something with one hand and take it back with the other as usual'. There was a stunned silence in the room and all eyes turned in my direction. Unknown to me, the man I was talking to was Vic Feather, General Secretary of the TUC. He had thought I was an official from the Bank of England. I hastily explained that I was a mere doctor and scientist, there to talk about space and nothing so important as the Budget

Peter Fairley came out to meet me and led me into Studio 2 (the main studio, Studio 1, was being used for the budget broadcast) and said he wanted to do a little face-to-face interview. We did so, and thanks to the studies I had done I was able to explain about the effects on the astronauts of the conditions and the tension they were enduring and explain why rescue was impossible. Even if a spare ship had been standing by, we could never catch up with a spacecraft on its outward journey.

This supposedly off-camera interview seemed to go well, and Peter asked me to hang on in case there was a newsflash and I would be needed to do an update. Unknown to both of us, however, Nigel Ryan, the Editor, was sitting on the top floor watching it all on a bank of TV monitors. Having liked the interview, he had got on to ITV and persuaded the network to take it as a 'space special'.

David Nicholas (then deputy Editor) said he would piece together a team of experts from different disciplines and make a programme. The excellent Alistair Burnett was the anchorman and the other two guests were Peregrine Worsthorne and Douglas Bader. Peter and I were there to commentate on medicine and science.

In the event that programme did not finish until four in the morning, by which time the astronauts had swung around the Moon and were on their way back to Earth. In the end Peter and I co-presented, taking it in turns to answer questions from Burnett. I would be asked how the astronauts were feeling, what they would be thinking about and how their training would have prepared them, and thanks to all the work I'd done in this field I was able to come up with some sensible answers.

Finally David Nicholas shook my hand and asked me to stay on the next morning. We had been bringing in eleven and a half million viewers!

After that I became a regular on space programmes for the rest of the Apollo series, which was enormously successful (with the sole exception of the ill-fated number 13 of course). I learned a great deal about presenting science on TV from Peter Fairley. He explained the knack of simplifying descriptions for the lay viewer: 'At ITN we don't talk about subsystems' he said. We had some prominent guest astronauts, including Jim Irwin, the first astronaut to ride on the Lunar Rover on the Apollo 15 mission. He was a very interesting man to talk to, and I learned so much from his personal accounts of working on the surface of the Moon.

With the NASA experts we had been looking at ways of allowing astronauts to explore a little further from the mother ship. We looked at ways of adding oxygen to their backpacks, and contributed to the increasing range of the EVA periods; in all the Apollo astronauts spent 22 hours on the lunar surface.

Towards the middle of the space programme I reluctantly decided to sell my Piper Colt. The Air Registration Board needed to carry out a mandatory inspection, and that would require removal of the special plastic fabric skin from fuselage, wings rudder and tailfin. After inspection it would need to be re-skinned at my expense. I pleaded with them to recognise the fact that the finest aircraft engineers at RAE could inspect to the required standards using equipment which would avoid removing the panels. My argument was not accepted, and I feared that the cost of having the skins replaced by the Piper Company in the States would be prohibitive. The aircraft engineers and technicians at the RAE Doping Department even offered to re-skin the aeroplane, but that wasn't accepted either. Reluctantly I was forced to sell the little Colt to a Flying Club which was prepared to take on the expense.

I got over my disappointment by buying a simply beautiful Bentley S3 in maroon, with Dolby Surroundsound and a host of other luxury features. That became my new baby, and it filled the gap created by the loss of the Colt.

It was a tremendous joy when in 1971 Kirstie moved down from Scotland and took a post at Sunningdale Preparatory School as Assistant Matron. She was now within striking distance of Farnborough and we were able to enjoy evenings out to the local pubs and have happy dinners at the nearby hotels. We got together as often as we could. She moved closer still when she took up the offer of a job with Mowlem in Bracknell, and our relationship became even stronger.

I took Kirstie along to ITN whenever I was taking part in a space special programme, and she got to know most of the staff there. She would stay and watch the programmes from the wings and meet the visiting astronauts and news presenters after the programme ended. They were all very welcoming and kind to her. Di Edwards-Jones, the lovely Welsh lady who directed News at Ten, had warned them to be on their best behaviour. 'Listen everyone' she said, 'Gordon's bringing a girlfriend and I don't want anyone to use the 'F' word.' Reggie Bosanquet's response was 'That's rich coming from you – you're the only one here who uses that kind of language'. The people in the studio collapsed with laughter, knowing, of course, that Bosanquet could well compete with her in his use of ripe language.

In the end everyone heeded Diana's request, and when Kirstie was present I rarely heard bad language coming from the control room. Our visits to ITN continued and our relationship flourished. It was wonderful to be able to take my girlfriend to the various functions we had in the Officers' Mess, and she got to know my colleagues and their wives well. Everyone, without exception, welcomed her to the Institute and the Farnborough social scene.

At that time, IAM was beginning to take space medicine more seriously and I was made an RAF Consultant in Aviation Medicine. I was also invited to write a textbook on Aviation Medicine (published later, in 1978) and was appointed as the Royal College of Physicians Reader (later Associate Professor) to the Diploma Course in Aviation Medicine. Then, as if I did not have enough on my plate, the Medical Branch suggested that I might be interested in taking an unusual dual post based at RAF North Luffenham as Commanding Officer of the AMTC, but continuing as a Consultant with research commitments and continue with my academic input at IAM as the Associate Professor. It was all go then, and I jumped at the chance to take on these responsibilities. I also started to make plans for the future.

Kirstie and I got engaged at the Queens Hotel in Farnborough on 15th June 1972. We began to make plans for our wedding later in the year, and of course the honeymoon.

We looked at all types of venues and exotic honeymoon spots, but an order from the Director General of Medical Services (DGMS) necessitated a swift change of plans. The DGMS told me I would be needed for an important NATO Exercise in Stornoway on the Scottish Isle of Lewis. It was scheduled to take place in the first few weeks of September - bang in the middle of our planned honeymoon period - and there was simply no way round it. That was an order that had to be obeyed and another examples of the 'exigencies of the Service'.

I phoned the Medical Branch and managed, unbelievably, to get through to the DGMS himself. 'Take your new wife with you' he said breezily. 'Put her up in the local hotel. And by the way, your promotion to the rank of Wing Commander will take effect while you are in the middle of the exercise.'

With that he rang off. I didn't know how I was going to tell Kirstie, but she took the news very well. She said she too had caused quite a stir in the family when she told her mother that we had to get married by a certain date. This was simply to meet the deadline for qualifying for a Commanding Officer's quarter at Luffenham, but her mother imagined there was another reason for the urgency! Kirstie had to convince her that that she was not pregnant, and eventually the flap it caused in the family calmed down.

As per our modified plans, our wedding took place on the 19th of August 1972 in the little Scottish Episcopal Church in Fortrose, attended by relatives, friends and colleagues from IAM. Don Cameron was my best man, his daughters were Kirstie's bridesmaids and his son Andrew was a pageboy, resplendent in his Highland outfit.

A quick honeymoon in Scotland in gorgeous August weather was followed by a dash over to Stornoway for the

NATO exercise. We put up at a small hotel in the town of Stornoway, within easy reach of the airport where the exercise was taking place. Kirstie managed to hire a car – well, a kind of a car - it had hopeless brakes and a gearbox that sometimes did or did not engage. It was almost a wreck and in my view was not really roadworthy. With the huge influx of service personnel into Stornoway there had been a run on cars for hire, and the one we got was about the last one left - and when I saw it I wasn't surprised no one else had hired it. But it did allow both of us to see quite a bit of the Isle of Lewis when the NATO exercise permitted.

I hadn't managed to take my fishing rods with me on the exercise, although the young Medical Officer with me in the Medical Centre had brought his and had found a small loch near the airfield which he decided to fish. I joined a bunch of locals who were leaning over a fence and watching him flogging away without apparently getting so much as a rise. The locals kept asking if he was having any luck. I understood their mild amusement the following day when the 'loch' turned out to be nothing more than a field that had flooded after a heavy downpour of rain a few days before our arrival!

As promised by the Director General of Medical Services, my promotion to the rank of Wing Commander came through and we were able to celebrate and round off the NATO exercise in an appropriate way. As an experience it was useful and interesting, but as a honeymoon venue it wasn't quite the same as Copacabana Beach.

In September 1972, I returned to RAF North Luffenham, this time as Commanding Officer of the AMTC. I was now able to make my own impact on the training there, assisted by my team of doctors, RAF GD Officers and Warrant

Officer and NCO technical and support staff. There was Moran Hughes as my deputy, who with Bill Smith, Ernie Jamieson and Ron Pearson, formed the mainstay of the aeromedical team. Gerry Murphy, a Royal Australian Air Force exchange officer, joined us, and he was later replaced by a fellow Australian, Greg Herring. I couldn't have asked for a better team if I had tried, and they were all enthusiastic about improving the standards of training at the Centre.

Shortly after I arrived we had a visit from Princess Margaret, and the then Station Commander was desperate to impress our royal visitor in every way he could. He had been briefed by MoD that she chain-smoked Lucky Strike cigarettes, and he actually arranged for someone to follow her with an ashtray, just in case it was needed!

Preparations went on for weeks before the visit, and it was difficult for my team to continue with the training courses for the hordes of aircrew that were now coming through the Centre. We were ordered to follow the old RAF tradition that 'if it doesn't move, paint it'.

It has to be said that on the day, the Station looked most impressive, and the visit turned out to be a success. Only one thing marred it for me. The astronaut Dick Gordon, who had flown on Apollo 12, had given me a 'space pen' after I gave him tips on winners during a visit with ITN to Sandown Park. He was most insistent that I should accept it in exchange for his winnings. The Station Commander borrowed it so that HRH could sign the Mess visitors' book with it, and I never saw it again; someone filched it. I was very fond of that pen and was extremely annoyed when it disappeared.

Otherwise the visit was successful. Princess Margaret was

interested in the work of the Centre and enjoyed watching through the observation windows of the chamber as the pilots attending the Course underwent rapid decompression.

By now Kirstie was heavily pregnant with our firstborn, and this gave rise to speculation by visiting aircrew that it was most likely to be a daughter (a 'slotted job' rather than a 'toggle job', in RAF slang). There had been a rumour among aircrew that wives of high-altitude flyers exposed to lower levels of oxygen always had daughters. I believe the rumour became so strong that John Ernsting had been asked to look at it. He found no sign that it was true, yet it persisted. Bets were on that in view of the time I spent at simulated altitude in our chambers our first child was certain to be a 'slotted job;' as it turned out, that theory certainly didn't hold up in my case. Our first two children were boys, conceived and born at a period of my career when I was hardly ever out of decompression chambers. Our eldest son, named Russell after his grandfather, was born in 1973, followed by William ('Willie') in 1976. For many years the rumour persisted and the next addition to our family was Melanie our daughter in 1979. To complete our family a third son, Alastair, was born in 1980. I never heard whether that did anything to throw doubt on the validity of the rumour, but I believe some bets were lost by a few of my colleagues and friends.

My involvement in space and the Apollo programme continued. While I was at AMTC I managed to fit in visits to the Manned Spacecraft Centre in Houston Texas. It was good to see that the RAF and IAM were now encouraging much more work in the field of space medicine. I used every opportunity on my visits to look for ideas and techniques that might benefit conventional aviation medicine and help with the training role of the Centre. I was particularly interested, among other things, in NASA's techniques for monitoring the wellbeing of astronauts during spaceflight and looked in detail at the medical and other monitoring stations in Mission Control.

I had a slightly difficult moment while out on one of these visits to the Manned Space Centre. It was just before one of the Apollo broadcasts, and ITN asked if I could send a short piece back by satellite to ITN House if the opportunity presented itself. It did, and I prepared a short presentation for recording back in ITN Studios in London. The intention was to use it for News at Ten the following night.

The floor manager had just cued me into my opening lines when I became aware of frantic waving by an agitated chap standing in the wings of the studio. Through a mix-up in allocation of the studio I had been broadcasting to CBC in Toronto!

I never found out if my piece went out live to the Canadian audience or even if it was used at all, but having missed the slot for transmission the poor CBC presenter had to retreat with his tail between his legs and the prospect of a wigging from his bosses.

Soon came the final Apollo mission, Apollo 17, which signalled an end to the programme. It was of particular interest to me, as John and I and the Division had been involved in calculating the distances to which an astronaut could safely explore on the surface of the Moon away from the mother craft. That distance had been stretched by the introduction of the Lunar Rover. As the programme unfolded and the geological exploration got more and more exciting, NASA agreed to allow an extension of the time the two astronauts could spend away from the Lunar Module. I hadn't taken account of this last-minute decision when making my calculations and I was a little anxious.

The Lunar Buggy had been damaged on the way out, and if it broke down the lives of the astronauts would be in danger, as their oxygen supply would not be sufficient to allow them to walk back to the spacecraft. Fortunately, the buggy behaved perfectly and the astronauts returned safely to the craft- but it was a near thing, and I was thankful it was over.

My involvement with space was not quite finished, however. In 1975 I was asked to join the space team at ITN for the Apollo/Soyuz link up. The anchorman again was Reggie Bosanquet, and I was joined by Geoff Perry, the physics master at Kettering Grammar School. He was a delightfully eccentric character and he and his pupils monitored all rocket launches in the world, particularly tracking Russian space activities with their homemade radio receivers.

The Apollo/Soyuz mission was launched without a hitch, with the aim of docking a US craft and a Russian craft together. Geoffrey Perry and the Kettering lads had calculated that the two spacecraft would come together over Bognor Regis. Here the handshake between the astronauts and cosmonauts would take place. He announced this during our programme, and the Mayor of Bognor urged car drivers to put on their headlights and householders to blaze their domestic lights as a salute. Unfortunately the Reuters news agency also picked up the fact that the docking would take place over the English coast, which spread the news to the world. Reportedly the Russians were not happy about this, as it seemed to favour the West and America's allies too much – at least, that was the rumour. The Russians vetoed the plan and the docking took place slightly later, when the two spacecraft were over Metz in France.

Reggie Bosanquet thought this was hysterical, and was longing to say that the Russians had in effect said 'bugger Bognor', echoing the phrase said to have been uttered by King George V on his death bed. Sadly, David Nicholas overruled him and to my knowledge the phrase was never broadcast.

While I was at AMTC, the BBC's Science Correspondent, James Burke, paid a visit to the Centre. His style was very different from that of Peter Fairley at ITN, although I had never actually been able to watch him on the BBC space programmes as they were on at the same time as ours from ITN. James asked if we could put something together for a programme on people exposed to extremes of endurance. He wanted to know what happened if pressure was lost in an aircraft or spacecraft.

I demonstrated this on TV using our chambers at the Centre. Of course I went a slate-blue colour and passed out. Unfortunately Kirstie and my mother (who was staying with us at the time) saw the programme and were in floods of tears when they saw me getting bluer in the face, talking gibberish and beginning to collapse. I'm afraid I had not been too open with them about the dangers of these experiments, and I got a maternal lecture on my responsibilities as a married man. We put the demonstration on tape and I believe it was used for years in teaching and other demonstrations, although I was never able to retrieve a copy for myself. Just as well perhaps, for the topic was never raised again in our household.

My unusual dual role was working well, and I enjoyed the link with IAM, where I could continue research and development work there with the applied work of training at AMTC, though on the downside, it did mean regular trips up and down the A1 between the two places. On one of these visits to IAM, the most unusual thing happened as I was driving down the A1. My Bentley's radiator started to blow steam, and I was forced to pull into a layby near Sandy in Bedfordshire. I peered into the engine and spotted the problem. A hoseclip had snapped and I was out of cooling liquid.

Suddenly I was surrounded by a group of about eight Hells Angels on powerful motorbikes.

'Heving a little trouble with the Roller, old chep?' they mocked.

'Yes I bloody well am' I said. 'It's a Bentley and right now I wish I had a Triumph Thunderbird like yours.'

That changed the mood entirely. I was invited to inspect and admire every one of their machines. The leader, a huge muscular chap in full riding leathers, jumped on his bike and flagged down an old couple who were trying to have a quiet day out in their car. They were ordered to take me to a garage further up the road, and we were given a motorcycle escort to make sure we got there.

The garage owner gasped in astonishment and horror at the spectacle. He was ordered to take me back down the road in his repair truck.

'That lot are notorious' he whispered. 'There will be

nothing left of your car after they are finished with it'. But he was wrong. The Bentley was intact, and actually being guarded by the other Hells Angels.

When the recovery was all sorted out, I thanked my new-found friends for their help and asked the garage owner to fill up their petrol tanks at my expense.

'You're OK mate' said the leader in gratitude. 'And if you ever want anyone sorted out, just give us a call.' I wasn't quite sure what he meant. At that moment I could think of several people that might be included in the offer, but needless to say I never had occasion to seek their services again.

I began to focus all my attention and energy into finalising the monitoring and training work I had started on my previous posting. With the help of the team, I increased the scope of the lectures and brought in new training techniques. We even had an ejection seat trainer to teach the crew to use the right posture to avoid back injury. We also trained them to deal with parachute dragging – if a pilot was dragged by the wind along the ground, he could easily suffer injuries to elbows and knees.

In 1974, a spatial disorientation familiarisation device was installed, with the purpose of demonstrating to aircrew the most common vestibular illusions and visual disturbances that can occur in flight. It was essentially a cab fitted with instruments and displays mounted on a turntable and it proved highly popular with the pilots.

Most of all I wanted to make major changes to the monitoring of aircrew during the rapid decompression phase. Through my NASA experiences at Houston, I believed that each aspect of monitoring had to be focused on separately.

One monitoring doctor just couldn't look at everything, and I felt this was a mistake and meant too much input to cope with. I therefore got the technicians to construct a new monitoring room, modelled on and looking remarkably like a miniature version of the one I had studied at Mission Control. Each monitoring doctor sat in front of a bank of television monitors presented with cameras focused on the pilot in the chamber and displays of records of heart rate, electrocardiograph and breathing parameters. It worked well, and despite the good-natured 'we have lift-off!' jokes, all the staff agreed that the monitoring and care of the pilot was much safer than before.

Despite the hectic life in North Luffenham and the travelling up and down the A1 between it and Farnborough, I still found time to bring up my young family and have a little fun at the same time. Every officer on the Station was expected to undertake a secondary duty. With my interest in motor racing and cars, I chose to set up a go-kart club, using bales of straw to mark the track and act as buffers. The karts were very simple, but it was great fun and quickly caught on. I remember we had a chap called Bruno Ferrari, a fruit merchant in London, who true to his name was a very fast driver and kept winning.

When the Director General of Medical Services (DGMS) announced that he wished to visit the Centre, he was somewhat put out to find that the Station Commander would not give him permission to land his own aircraft there because the go-kart track was in the way! He had to divert to nearby RAF Wittering and be driven up in a staff car. He wasn't amused at this, and when he arrived on the Station I think he made his feelings known to the Station Commander.

I had not been informed of the reason for the visit by DGMS and wondered what had prompted this unusual departure from his busy schedule. It had to be something pretty important, I thought. It wasn't long before the reason came out. To my astonishment and great delight he informed me that I was to be awarded the coveted Richard Fox Linton Memorial Prize for my contribution to flight safety. To me this was a recognition of the work which everyone at the Centre had contributed to in building up AMTC and setting the standard of training that went on there. I considered that although I was receiving this award I was accepting it on behalf of every member of the Team who had supported me so magnificently.

In the summer of 1976, John Ernsting was made deputy Head of Research at IAM, a senior appointment which carried substantial administration and research supervisory duties. I was asked to return to Farnborough and act as his deputy. We left our married quarter in Luffenham and after a short spell in a married quarter in Beverley Crescent, we bought and moved into a lovely house in Farnham. It sat on top of the hill which was said to be the very spot from which Dean Swift had looked down on distant farmworkers two hundred and fifty years before and thought up the idea of Gulliver's Travels and a world populated by miniature people.

Our daughter Melanie was born on 18th May 1979 in the Cambridge Military Hospital in Aldershot. With the family getting larger and another baby (Alastair) on its way, I had to do major DIY in our house to create enough rooms to bring up our new family. By the time young Alastair arrived into the world on 11th July 1980, I had just managed to complete the house reconstruction project and a brand new nursery bedroom was waiting and ready for him.

Unfortunately my mother didn't live to see his arrival. She died from a heart attack on the 6th of January 1980, having had a whale of a time over the Christmas and New Year festivities when she had danced eightsome reels until the wee small hours. What a way to go!

The two older boys missed their grandma terribly, and Kirstie and I missed the sense of fun she had brought on every one of her visits to us in Farnham.

I now needed to put my love of classic sports cars aside, and bought a VW Camper Van. It turned out to be a most useful purchase, acting as a 'mobile nappy-changing vehicle', and was great for holidays and perfect for moving our young family around. What a comedown it was from the luxury cars I had enjoyed! But family needs had to take priority over hobbies and we had to adapt.

I was now heavily engaged in lecturing to doctors on the ten-month course for the Diploma of Aviation Medicine, and was getting little or no time for any research projects. With my previous exposure on national television I was still receiving invitations to broadcast and lecture, and the RAF encouraged me to accept them, as they saw it as good publicity for the Service. I took part in BBC programmes like *The World At One* and contributed to several broadcasts from Bush House for the BBC overseas service, about in-flight emergencies and ejection seat escape.

I was also invited to give a Royal Society of Medicine Children's Christmas Lecture. While I was there, my samples of space food (candy bars for inside the astronauts' helmets) were filched. I knew it had been the wee lad in the front row, because when I announced that the person who had eaten the candy bars would probably get dreadful stomach ache I saw his face turn a greyish-green colour. It wasn't true of course - they were perfectly edible - but I hoped it might teach him a lesson for the future.

My lecturing and presenting commitments continued. I lectured in schools and university departments, presenting the work of IAM and Space Medicine to aviation groups and various medical societies, and of course I loved doing it. Perhaps I got carried away, but I seriously wondered if this might be leading to a change in career.

I confided in David Nicholas (now the Editor of ITN) that I was thinking that I might like to become a science and medicine correspondent. Peter Fairley had left ITN by that time and I knew David was toying with the idea of building up a science and medicine team for ITN. He was taken aback by my suggestion and thought that it would be mad for me to give up a successful career. But generously, he gave me the opportunity to taste the TV presenter's life as an ITN space, science and medicine correspondent.

He arranged for Tyne Tees Television to let me loose on a live broadcast. A surgeon had discovered that pressure suits (based on the type used by RAF pilots) helped in the treatment of shock after a coronary thrombosis. Tyne Tees wanted to use this story for a magazine slot after the news, so I was despatched up to Newcastle for the programme. The RAF Medical Branch and the MoD were delighted to have me do this, as recruitment to the Medical Branch was down and the publicity was welcomed.

For a second time I met my old friend Arthur Ferns, the

chap whose MG I had run into when we were students at Glasgow University. We chatted and reminisced for ages on the platform of Newcastle Railway Station and I lost all sense of time. I had to make a frantic dash up to the studios and only just arrived as the programme started, so my equipment was not fully prepared. I demonstrated one of the suits, but having blown it up I found I could not reach the valve to dump the pressure. Fortunately one of the floor staff realised I was in trouble and hit the valve.

David Nicholas was complimentary about my performance, but still expressed doubt about my thoughts for such a major change of career direction. He went to the trouble of paying me a visit in Farnborough, when he pointed out that as a medical broadcaster I would be expected to churn out articles for newspapers and magazines to get well known. Still, he very kindly gave me another opportunity to look at the world of television news broadcasting by inviting me to give the annual lecture in memory of Richard Spriggs, an ITN reporter who tragically lost his life aboard a motor launch during the ITV coverage of Cowes Week. His parents were in the audience, and my talk about the future of space travel seemed to go well.

Afterwards I met up with David and told him again how much I had enjoyed the experience and how I still wanted to become a medicine and science correspondent. Again he expressed his worry that it might not be sensible to throw up a lifetime of work and achievement. He knew I would have to start from the very beginning and was trying to put me off the idea in the nicest possible way. In the end he admitted the decision had to be mine.

To try and unclutter my mind and help with the decision,

I went back to my touchstone, Cody's tree at Farnborough. The branch I had ascribed to broadcasting seemed to peter out half way up, but the central branch - the medical and science branches - went straight up to the top and seemed to twirl around in a sort of crown shape. A portent? As a scientist I really shouldn't entertain such ideas, but I have always had a slight superstitious streak.

I realised then that any major change of direction at my stage of life would be a reckless move, and put the idea to one side. I think David was relieved when I told him, but he promised that whenever the opportunity arrived ITN would always be delighted to have me on as a guest presenter.

The major part of my work was now administration, and despite my role in teaching and training doctors in aviation medicine, which I enjoyed, I still felt unsettled. There were changes happening at the Institute which we all disliked. Cuts in staff and facilities meant a revamp of some of the Divisions and Sections. As part of the changes I was made Head of the Altitude Division, taking over from John Ernsting, and although I enjoyed being able to run my own projects and those of the Sections within the Division, it did create more administration. I was not particularly fond of that.

To make matters worse, JE went off on sabbatical year to the US Air Force School of Aviation Medicine (SAM) in the States, where he worked on OBOGS (On Board Oxygen-Generating Systems) for aircraft. I greatly missed him as a mentor. I took over some of his committee work, like chairing meetings and supervising the work of the Sections. Dr Alastair Macmillan and his team helped me enormously in this, but it was still pretty demanding stuff. I tried to get on with my teaching programme, but there was little or no time for research projects. I missed that side of the work and began to feel there was a sense of loss of direction at the Institute. The Cold War was now beginning to lose its grip, and with the final triumph of Apollo 17, the Apollo/Soyuz link and the Skylab programme, interest in manned space flight was pretty much over.

I began searching around for new fields that I could get my teeth into. I talked at length to my friend and colleague Moran Hughes, who had supported me so well as my deputy at AMTC. Before coming into the Medical Branch of the Service, Moran had been a doctor with Unilever, and he had great experience of the work of an Industrial Health Medical Officer. He saw a bright future in the field of occupational medicine, yet I still couldn't decide where to go or what to do next.

I went back and looked at the life of Samuel Cody. He had not stopped after his major achievement in powered flight, but had begun to wonder how he could use what he had learned in the real world. He had looked at the possibility of flying passengers in an aeroplane – quite unheard of at that time - and even converted one of his craft into an air ambulance, with stretchers, doctors and equipment aboard to pick up injured people from inaccessible places like battlefields and get them to hospital quickly.

Cody was applying all the information he had gained about design, testing and flying aircraft and using what he had learned for the public good. It finally dawned on me that rather than keeping to the narrow world of aviation and space flight, I should be doing the same thing. That had to be my new goal, and my talks with Moran Hughes seemed to point in the direction of occupational medicine. The question was - what skills and expertise could I bring to this new specialty?

I found the answer in a most bizarre way. One day I was queuing for a quick snack in Waterloo Station before catching my train back to Farnborough. I was looking at the bill of fare, which was illustrated by luridly-coloured photos showing the range of burgers offered for sale. At the top they were offering a new 'Super Mega Whopperburger' or something of that kind, which seemed to have layer upon layer of meat, cheese, salad, mayonnaise and so on. The chap in front of me asked the young lad behind the counter how the 'Whopperburger' differed from his usual previous version. Both, he said, looked the same. The answer came back that they had changed the content and it now included three extra layers.

The chap in the queue shook his head. 'That's three layers too many for me, those extras would do nothing for my weight problem' he said, pointing to his large, protruding stomach. I nodded in agreement, and as I did so the penny dropped. Somewhere in my head a light bulb flashed. I had had a Eureka moment; I had just spotted a new way of using my skills and experience in aerospace medicine for the common good.

His remark reminded me that it was normal procedure in the RAF that when a new aeroplane came into service or changed its operational role, test pilots put the aircraft through its paces. Using their skills and techniques they define a 'flight envelope' ensuring that the aircraft systems meet all requirements and operational demands. Likewise we, as aviation doctors, use our skills and experience to define an 'operational envelope' within which the human systems can cope with every demand. Not only that but flight envelopes often have to be changed to meet requirements of the Service, and as the man in the burger shop had noticed, albeit in a different context, even the smallest change can tip a previously safe and healthy situation into a hazardous one. In other words, it is important not only to define the 'safety envelopes' but to constantly check and recheck them looking for changes that might have safety implications. Was this the answer I had been looking for?

If we could combine the skills and experience of the test pilot with the aerospace doctor, we might be able to define 'safe operating envelopes' and improve the safety and wellbeing of those engaged in thousands of different tasks carried out in hundreds of everyday occupations. I was certain that no work of this type was being carried out in the field of occupational medicine. The man in front of me in the queue had just handed the answer to me –on a plate as it were!

I was sure now that I could produce a new research protocol that we could use to the benefit of the public good. So excited was I with the idea that I quite forgot about my lunch and rushed back to my laboratory at IAM.

How bizarre, I thought, that a simple observation in a burger bar could possibly open up a new career pathway. Then I recalled how a distant relative of mine, James Watt, had watched a kettle boil in his mother's kitchen. That simple observation gave him the idea to modify and make more efficient the existing Newcomen steam engines. It was a massive contribution to industry and engineering, and using the good old RAF 'Mark One Eyeball' had made it possible. Could history be repeating itself?

The next step was to try to find a job where I could develop my ideas of applying my skills for the common purpose. I looked at several possibilities, but none seemed right. Universities had little or no research in this area, and medical posts in Industrial Medicine (the predecessor of Occupational Medicine) were only to be found in major heavy industries, where most of the work-related health problems had already been addressed. True, there was exceptionally high-quality research being carried out at the Institute of Occupational Medicine (IOM) in Edinburgh, and I wondered about joining them. But when I looked into what they might offer, I felt they were much too National Coal Board-focused for my purposes.

In the end, I decided to bide my time until just the right opening came along, one where I could start to put my theories into practice. Eventually I found it, but not quite in the way I had envisioned. I was not to know that when the opportunity did come, it would have momentous consequences for my life.

CHAPTER NINE

BY ROYAL APPOINTMENT

The next turn in my career was an extraordinary one. It began with an advertisement in the British Medical Journal in the autumn of 1981, announcing that a small medical practice was looking for a doctor up in Caithness. Based in the tiny village of Canisbay, close to John O'Groats and almost as far north in Britain as you can get, it was a single-handed dispensing practice looking after a handful of farm workers and villagers.

You might ask why on earth a chap like me in middle age with a young family and a well-established career in aviation medicine would want to move six hundred miles to the back of beyond, but somehow it felt right. I reasoned that it would be an ideal platform from which to complete my plans for occupational medicine research and get them written up. It would not be too demanding, and it would help me to brush up on clinical medicine. It would also be a good opportunity to start concentrating on writing articles, papers and perhaps another textbook – this time not on aviation but on occupational medicine.

I mentioned the job to Kirstie, confident that she would dismiss the idea as out of the question, but she said she was prepared to consider it as she felt it would be good opportunity to be nearer her elderly parents now living in Strathpeffer, near Inverness. With Kirstie's backing I filled in an application, a somewhat half-baked and fairly brief one I think, and forgot about it.

Then some weeks later, in the December, I received an invitation to go up to Inverness for an interview. I took the night sleeper train, arriving on a bitterly cold Tuesday morning. I was frozen stiff as I emerged from the station and felt the blast of cold from a Highland winter.

I had to kill some time looking round the Inverness shops until it was time for the interview, which was held in an old building down by the river. The panel (none of whom I knew) asked me all kinds of questions, including some rather odd ones; one elderly tweed-clad lady asked, 'Do you have any horses for stabling?' I said no, and she asked, 'But you ride?' Yes, I said, but I wasn't really a horseman. 'But you were a member of the Cavalry Club?' she said. That was true, but the information had not been on my form. I was beginning to get the feeling that this job, simple as it had seemed, was not as straightforward as I had imagined. They explained that they were not sure how long the practice would continue independently, as being just a one-doctor practice it might well be merged with another. I said I was really only thinking about it as an interim measure, so that was fine.

Then came the crucial information. 'You do know that one of the commitments of the practice is to look after the Castle of Mey?'

Now I knew why they had looked into my background so carefully. The Castle of Mey, just a few miles east of Canisbay, was the private holiday residence of the Queen Mother. Built in the 16th century, it had been purchased by her in a semi-derelict condition in 1952, following the death of her husband, King George VI, and she had fully restored it. She was using it as a holiday retreat, but frequently visited Longhoe Farm on her estate, where she loved to be among her pedigree sheep and cattle. The job did not appear to entail any contact with Her Majesty, but it did mean looking after the staff and estate workers at the castle.

I was offered the job pretty much on the spot and took it without hesitation, although my colleagues thought I was crazy to go all the way up to the far north of Scotland to work in general practice. One of them gave me a book called *Trout and how to catch them*, assuming I would have little else to do in my new home. Indeed the practice was tiny, with hardly enough work to keep even one man busy, but my late mother had given away most of my father's rods and reels after he died and inadvertently included my own decent rods and tackle with them.

Of course I could not walk into general practice without a refresher, so I shadowed our own GP in Farnborough for about two months before taking up the appointment, learning about the latest developments in medication and so on.

We moved up with the family in March 1982. It was appalling weather with horizontal rain, a depressing welcome to Caithness. We stayed in a local hotel until we were able to move into a Health Board house with surgery and dispensary attached.

We had great help in settling in from Jackie Pyle, the

previous doctor's wife. He was in Saudi doing a medical detachment, and Jackie was a great help with Kirstie and our young family. She was a godsend to me, helping me with dispensing from the practice. I also appreciated her local knowledge, and she was great at giving directions to find patients in some of the most remote crofts and farms.

Most of the work was pretty routine and much as you would expect from a small general practice. There were plenty of overseas visitors to John o' Groats, and communication with foreign visitors was difficult at times. Fortunately my Range Rover, bought just before taking on the practice, helped to get me to places which were almost impossible to reach with anything but a four by four. I used it on one occasion as an 'ambulance' to pick up an overseas visitor who had been taken ill while camping out in a remote and difficult-to-access area. It was a very versatile vehicle indeed.

One unusual job we had was looking after people who had cycled in a variety of two and three-wheeler bicycles from Land's End to John O'Groats; some of them were arriving practically welded to their bikes. The district nurse and I had to deal with some of the most appalling saddle sores you could ever imagine!

I had not been up there long when we had a visit to our house from Sir Ralph Anstruther, the Queen Mother's Equerry Treasurer, and Martin Leslie, the Factor at Balmoral. Clearly they wanted to make sure I was a suitable man for a position that would bring me so close to Her Majesty. It was clear that they had checked everything about us. When they arrived Kirstie was boiling lobsters which had been specially caught and given to us by a grateful crofter patient, but despite the unwelcoming state of the kitchen and the rest of the house it was a delight to meet them both.

Although I had never met Sir Ralph before, I felt that I knew him from watching him on television placing a wreath on the Cenotaph on behalf of the Queen Mother on Remembrance Sunday. Martin Leslie I had also never met before. He was the son of a friend of my mother's whom I had met at parties during my leave periods. The pair were visiting the castle to get it ready for Her Majesty's visit, although Sir Ralph joked that the real reason was Martin Leslie's fondness for 'Caribbean cake', a speciality bake of Mrs Webster, the resident housekeeper at Mey.

I later understood why the Queen Mother held Martin Leslie in such high regard. He had been commanded by Her Majesty to represent her at a memorial service for the late Reverend Bell, Minister of Canisbay Church, who had died just after my arrival. Mr Leslie lent such a 'presence' to the service that at times you could almost believe that Her Majesty was there in the royal pew herself. It was good to meet two such pleasant members of the Household, and I looked forward to working with them.

Many of the castle staff were elderly and needed regular treatment, so I agreed to hold regular surgeries at the castle, and said I would aim to be there at a certain time every day. On the first morning I turned into the approach road to the back courtyard to see Her Majesty's Range Rover and driver positioned at the main castle steps. I was met by her steward and butler, William Tallon, widely known as 'Backstairs Billy', who was warm and charming and very helpful. He invited me to follow him up to see Sir Martin Gilliatt and Sir Ralph Anstruther, the two Equerries to the Queen Mother.

'The Presence will be here shortly' they told me. An odd term, but it could only mean one thing. And a few moments later, that was exactly what I felt; a presence. Something changed in the room. Perhaps the two courtiers stiffened or there was a silence, but I knew immediately that Her Majesty was with us. I swung round to see that she had indeed entered the room.

I had been told I should address her initially as 'Your Majesty', bowing from the neck, then 'ma'am'. I hope I remembered this. She was friendly and gave me a warm welcome to the castle and to Caithness. She told me that the previous day she had been to open the new Kessock bridge, close to my mother's home in Inverness. 'We didn't see much of it because the mist was down' she said. After a few moments she smiled and turned away. That was to be the first meeting of many.

I soon began to settle into my duties at the castle. I would be told each day whether I had a quiet clinic or a busy clinic. Then one day Sir Martin advised me, 'The Queen will be taking the corgis for a walk in the Policies and will be pleased if you could join her'. This was a command of course, not a request to be accepted or refused. 'The Policies' was the term they used for the grounds of the castle.

Soon this became a fairly regular event while she was staying at the castle. I would be asked to meet her in the grounds, and we would walk through the Policies, talking of all kinds of things, though never anything to do with medicine. She liked to talk about her favourite roses and her gardener's tree planting programme. When we went for a walk on the beach path she would wear her blue mackintosh, wellington boots and a battered old fishing hat (she referred to it as an 'old friend'). I could always tell from her attire what I was in for. No matter the weather, driving rain and howling wind, she would relish her bracing walks and I was expected to enjoy them too. 'Nothing like it for blowing away the cobwebs' she would say encouragingly.

Then one day she stopped beside the wall to the garden. 'You know this wall is fifteen feet high,' she said out of the blue. 'It has to be fifteen, if it's any less the wind changes from one type of flow to another much more damaging one. But of course, you would know all about that sort of thing.'

That gave me something to think about. She was letting me know in her own way that she knew my background. It was well known that she liked flying and reputedly adored Concorde, having flown in and even taking the controls of that wonderful aircraft before it was commissioned. A few years later she asked for a flight to mark her 85th birthday, which took place on August 6 1985. She said that whenever Concorde passed over Clarence House, she would wave. From that moment on all Concorde pilots turned their landing lights on and flashed them when they flew over her home.

She had a grasp I wouldn't have believed possible of technical and scientific matters. It was clear that aircraft and flying were quite an interest of hers. She had made a visit to RAF St Athan in Glamorgan, where she had met a group of RAF apprentices who had made her a model of an old aircraft. We talked about the Queen's Flight, but her real preference was helicopters. Obviously she had heard about my previous work at Farnborough and had taken an interest. Equally obviously, the equerries were feeding her information.

One day I was getting out of my Range Rover when my coat caught against the pillar and I heard something snap. 'Bugger!' I said, in the hearing of William Tallon. 'I hope it's my leg and not my stethoscope.' He looked puzzled, until I explained that a broken leg would heal in about six weeks, but my stethoscope was irreplaceable, as I had had it since I had been a student. Unfortunately it was the stethoscope that had suffered; it had snapped at the bell and there was no way of repairing it. Billy must have told the Queen Mother about this incident, because I had a message that she had made enquiries about the condition of the Doctor's 'favourite stethoscope'.

Another story which apparently reached Her Majesty was an incident which I recounted to Sir Martin Gilliatt. It happened in 1961, just before my detachment to IAM Farnborough. One of the IAM Hunter Mk 4 aircraft had fuel pump failure on approach to landing. The pilot ejected at 400 feet unhurt, and the aircraft came to a crash landing on Tweseldown racecourse at the far end of the runway. When RAE asked the army unit responsible for maintaining the racecourse if a communicating gate could be opened so they could retrieve the Hunter, the army major responded, 'Not really the Hunter Chase Season old boy, but don't worry, we'll collect your chap in one of our horseboxes and get him back to you as soon as we can'. The Queen Mother and Sir Martin, both racing enthusiasts, loved that story and reputedly retold the tale several times at her dinner parties.

The Queen Mother had passed her 80th birthday when I joined the practice and although she was in marvellous health, this happy state of affairs was clearly not going to continue indefinitely. Sir Martin, was concerned about her health, particularly as she tended to refuse treatment and had a habit of dismissing a dose of flu as nothing more than a 'slight chill'. He had suggested that she might like to take one of the Queen's physicians with her up to Caithness, an idea which she had dismissed out of hand. But he persisted and got her round to the idea of accepting a Medical Officer to look after the health of her aging staff. With her concern for the health and wellbeing of her staff she readily agreed, much to the relief of the two equerries.

One day I had a phone call to say that one of the house guests had been taken seriously ill and had collapsed. Although I quickly understood that it was not the Queen Mother herself, I burned rubber along the four-mile road to the castle. I was ushered into one of the tower bedrooms, where the man in question was lying on the floor flat out and deeply unconscious. It was not at all obvious what was wrong.

I sent everyone away so that I could examine him in private. He was breathing, shallowly, and his pulse was thin and thready. I looked around, wondering what could have happened, and on the dressing table I spotted a half-eaten bar of chocolate. I guessed that he was diabetic and had passed into a coma, though I couldn't be 100 percent sure if it was hypoglycaemic (lack of sugar) or hyperglycaemic (lack of insulin). I plumped for the former as the most likely diagnosis and fortunately had a vial of glucose solution in my bag, which works almost instantaneously in a hypo case. He was beginning to fit, so I asked for help from Ruth, Baroness Fermoy, who as Woman of the Bedchamber was a close friend and confidante of the Queen Mother. She was of course Princess Diana's grandmother and proudly told me that she had been a VAD in the war and would be glad to assist me.

I asked her if she could help to keep the man still while I looked for a vein, and she physically pinned him down to the floor while I tried to give an injection. I found a vein and got the glucose in, and within a few minutes he was coming round and I got two pages to help lift him on to his bed. I was invited by Lady Fermoy to join her for a gin and tonic in the Queen Mother's drawing room. It was one of Backstairs Billy's usual lethal gin and tonics, I don't know the exact mixture but I suspect that it was something like five parts gin and one part tonic. But boy did I appreciate that drink.

The Queen Mother herself was not there, as she was, I believe, out on one of her annual expeditions to Hattie Munro's antique shop, the Ship's Wheel in Thurso. When she returned, Lady Fermoy left the drawing room to meet her at the main door and, I have no doubt, to tell her all about the goings-on she fortunately had missed. The Queen Mother came into the drawing room, smiled and said 'Thank you Doctor, don't let us keep you from your gin and tonic'. She said how grateful she was that I had reacted so promptly. Having ascertained from Ruth Fermoy that the house guest had recovered fully, she quickly steered the conversation away from health matters by showing me an antique telescopic toasting fork she had bought.

There I was sitting on HM's couch in the holy of holies and wondering how I could best make my exit. There was a very precise protocol around encounters with the Queen Mother. For example, she would let you know when it was time to leave by taking you to the window and inviting you to look at the view, saying, 'I think we can see the Orkneys today' (whether one could or not). The correct response was then to request that you take your leave, make a small bow of the head and walk backwards for a couple of steps. After one of 'Backstairs Billy's' extra strong gin and tonics I hoped

I would manage that last manoeuvre without the indignity of falling over. I did manage a dignified exit from the Presence, just!

I was puzzled at the unusual number of staff seeking medical consultations during my visits to the castle over the course of one particular week. It was the custom for Her Majesty to give the entire staff a day out for a picnic on Orkney Island. The only problem was that it meant a crossing by small ferry over the notorious Pentland Firth. On previous outings most of the staff had been seasick, and instead of looking forward to the day out in Orkney they dreaded the thought of the journey. Some sought a prescription for Quells to allay their seasickness, while others tried to avoid the outing on the grounds of a convenient bout of ill health. Being liable to seasickness myself I had every sympathy with their problem, but I was wary about prescribing medicine for this kind of situation. I resorted to handing out some of the practical measures we gave to RAF aircrew who had bailed out of a stricken aircraft over the ocean and had to survive in rubber dinghies. Whether my advice was taken or not I don't know, but nothing more about the picnic was heard and I noted that on the day of the outing the Pentland Firth was the calmest it had ever been in living memory. How thankful I was that I didn't finish up with the entire castle staff as patients, all completely out of action.

Then came a very difficult case. Her Majesty was worried about one of her employees and was seeking reassurance about his state of health. I got a direct order from Sir Ralph to seek the best specialist medical help. One of the RAF hospitals in England had just installed a CAT scanner (a new technology at the time) and I arranged for an RAF consultant physician I knew to see him. The outcome of his hospital attendance was good and it gave me the opportunity to put my new occupational medicine approach into action. I identified the problem - an additional duty - and it needed only slight modification to his working schedule to put things right.

The Queen Mother was greatly relieved, and she invited Kirstie and me to 'join us' one evening at a party at the neighbouring Castle of Keiss. It was owned by Dixie Miller, an influential American speaker and lecturer with whom she was very friendly. We found the event rather formal, with various bankers and business types who were all very nervous and understandably stiff. Sir Martin came over and took me to meet some of the guests, and I noticed that he introduced me to one of them as the Queen Mother's doctor, while to another I was introduced as 'our Wing Commander'. This was odd, particularly as service rank was used only for and by the very senior members of the household like the equerries, but I said nothing.

As time went on I was asked more and more to join her Majesty in the Policies. The conversation began to change from aviation and space to family matters. I was asked if I was happy in Caithness and how the family were getting on. There were cocktail parties with HM's own friends, and more and more I felt I was being treated as one of the household.

Then one day Sir Martin stopped me and said the Queen Mother was worried about the hordes of starlings which were getting into nearby Freswick Castle. She said the place ought to be lived in again, and perhaps it might be a suitable family home for me to buy. The birds were coming down the chimney into the old drawing room and making a mess of the place. We agreed to take a look, and Kirstie and I collected the key from the farmhouse close to the castle. It was the size of a pipe wrench!

The castle was like a scene from the Hammer House of Horror. When I pushed on the door it emitted a terrible creaking sound. The place was something of a white elephant, having been unlived in for some time and latterly used as a small restaurant which had failed. We inspected the rooms, and tried to picture ourselves living there and climbing up the steep spiral staircase to bed with only a rope handle to help us keep our balance. The views from the windows of the castle were spectacular, and from the great hall we looked down to the angry, foaming Pentland Firth. Any romantic notions of owning a castle were quashed by practical considerations. We really couldn't see ourselves living in that pile.

The final decision was made when we noticed that there was an eight foot by four foot patch of ground in the courtyard which we were told was not for sale, as someone was buried there. That finished it for Kirstie! We were definitely not going to live there.

Not long after this, Billy Tallon met me at the courtyard gate and asked me if I could meet with Sir Martin in the Equerry's room. When I walked in he addressed me as Wing Commander. This was only the second time he had used my Service rank, and it seemed suspiciously formal. I began to fear that I had committed some grave error of diplomacy, or been guilty of some terrible indiscretion.

'Do sit down, Dr Sharp' he said. 'I have the pleasure of informing you that I am commanded by Her Majesty to offer you the position of Physician Extraordinary to the Household at Mey.' He quickly added that it would, of course, mean I had 'access by the back stairs'.

You could have knocked me down with a feather. 'Have I been going up the wrong stairs?' I asked, utterly failing to grasp his message. 'No no!' said Sir Martin, smiling for the first time. 'Her Majesty likes to use archaic terminology, but what it means is she now considers you her personal physician at Mey. Granting access if required to the Queen's chambers in the castle is an ancient and quite unusual privilege.'

Of course I accepted, once I had picked myself up off the floor. This was indeed an exceptional honour. It was a personal honorific which was entirely at the Queen Mother's discretion, because the Castle of Mey was her own house.

Sir Martin went on to explain that I would not be part of the official Royal Medical Household of the Sovereign, which was the Lord Chamberlain's gift. This honorific was a unique and separate one which, to my amusement, came into the same category as her personal piper. I wondered if, had I persisted with learning the bagpipes at school, I might have been able to double up as doctor and piper to the Household!

In fact I later discovered that the arrangements for medical care for the Royal Family are very complex. The 'Medical Household' comprises a range of Physicians and Surgeons to the Sovereign and to the Royal Household, though none are anything like full-time. However the 'Apothecaries to the Household' at Windsor and London hold daily surgeries, while other Apothecaries receive small salaries. The Queen Mother's medical care is arranged entirely on a private basis, although whenever she is resident in London, Windsor, Sandringham and even Balmoral, her medical needs are taken care of by one of the Sovereign's appointed Apothecary/Physicians. The problem was that when she was at the Castle of Mey her health needs were not covered by such an arrangement, a worrying gap.

I still couldn't take in what had happened, but I was soon welcomed as a 'member' of the Household when Sir Martin handed me a personal letter from Sir Ralph Southward, the QM's physician/apothecary at Clarence House.

I was still puzzled about why the honorific had been bestowed for something which was essentially my job, and asked Sir Martin straight out why I had been so honoured.

'Well' he said, 'this has been an unusual year for us at the Castle and we have all been very grateful for the professional way you have looked after us all. Queen Elizabeth was touched by the sacrifices you made in your service career to help make our time at the Castle a happier and healthier one.'

How on earth could they have known that to take up the appointment to the practice in time for Her Majesty's visits to the Castle of Mey, I had missed out on my automatic promotion due in September of that year, with all the salary and pension implications? But know they did, and although I had mentioned this to nobody, the Household must have learned it from somewhere. I deduced that it must have come from my ex-Director General of Medical Services (DGMS), Sir David Atkinson. Not only that, he must have told them that I had been next in line to be the Whittingham Professor of Aviation Medicine. This was the one loss I did actually regret, and the Household seemed to be aware of it. The Professorship was crucial in many ways to giving me the continuity of academic status for my planned venture into occupational medicine research. It wasn't until some time later that I discovered that that sacrifice had not gone unnoticed either.

At first, I was very worried about whether I would be expected to remain in Caithness and continue with my commitments at the Castle of Mey. Although I enjoyed the work, it was not my final goal, and the position would totally put paid to all my plans for the future. I knew Kirstie had found it difficult to adapt to living in Caithness after the busy life of a serving officer's wife and the challenges of bringing up a family. She had tried to adapt by helping me out with some of the administrative work of the practice, and had started a little nursery group in the school next to our house. But I knew she was finding it hard going, and the prospect that we might have to remain in Canisbay was quite a formidable one.

I knew I had to get our life and my future work sorted out. I asked to see Sir Ralph Anstruther, who was taking a week's leave from his work at the Castle of Mey and using it as an opportunity to visit his mother and sister in their house in the nearby village of Watten. He invited Kirstie and me to join him and his mother for afternoon tea. He listened sympathetically and with understanding to my dilemma.

With the honorific, he assured me, there were no formal commitments whatsoever, and if I chose to continue with the practice there I would always be considered as part of the Household at Mey. If I continued in practice elsewhere, or sought a position where I could pursue my research, it would still be a great comfort to the senior Household members to know that I would be available for medical advice and assistance if required. This was just what I wanted to hear, and it came as an enormous relief.

Some time later I was delighted when Sir Martin told me that he had recently been 'in the Presence' and that Her

Majesty would be pleased to restore my former academic status as a titular Professor. With a smile on his face, he added that it would not be necessary for me to grow my hair long! This was a reference to a comment I had made that when I became the Associate Professor (Reader) in Aviation Physiology years before, my children hated the idea of having a 'long-haired nutty professor' as a father. The remark had obviously been passed on to Her Majesty – more evidence of how her staff acted as her eyes and ears.

With a new spring in my step, I set about the ongoing work of the practice and the regular visits to the Castle and continued to participate in the strange but fascinating life there. One of those delights was the Queen Mother's beloved annual Mey Games, put on in a small field adjacent to the Castle by the local branch of the Royal British Legion. They were simple and very basic, but they were great fun and the locals loved them. I believe they still do; these days they are held under the patronage of the Duke and Duchess of Rothesay. She asked if I was taking part in the tug of war, and although somewhat startled I felt I had to say I was. 'Or will you be on call?' she said with a meaningful smile. She was letting me know that she was happy to supply an excuse!

One of those who couldn't find a ready excuse not to take part was our neighbour the Rev. Alec Muir, minister of the local church in Canisbay, which HM regularly attended. Like me he had been approached to join the tug o' war team. He was a lightly-built man and knew he would be up against some of the huge, muscular immensely fit US Navy personnel from the nearby Forss Base. They usually fielded a much heavier team than we ever could from the Castle, even though ours included well-built members of the Royal Protection Squad.

At the last minute the Reverend found an excuse for opting out of the tug o' war event, but he nobly agreed to enter the greasy log competition (a kind of pillow fight conducted whilst straddling a greasy, slippery log). He was aching, bruised and slightly battered for days afterwards and the District Nurse and I had to treat him for the after-effects. As usual the games that year were a great success and the QM wandered around the field talking to the locals in a friendly and relaxed manner.

We never quite knew what was going to turn up at HM's games. In the middle of the piping events a coach with a bunch of American tourists pulled up at the entrance to the field and started to spill out into the grounds. At that time security around the members of the royal family was much more relaxed, but I saw the British Legion Organiser and the senior police officer with the Royal Protection Squad having a hastily-arranged conversation with the Queen Mother. On her instruction apparently, the coach party was admitted, and it was an amazing sight to see their faces as the QM welcomed them all in and engaged most of them in conversation. She even allowed photographs to be taken of them as a group standing next to her. That was something none of us was allowed to do, except on very rare or special occasions, and only with her express permission. The driver of the coach was in a complete daze - I don't think he had realised that the QM would be present at the games. His reputation, and I am sure the size of his tip from the coach party, would reflect the rare privilege that his passengers had enjoyed that afternoon.

Everyone, including I believe the Queen Mother, applauded Alec Muir's stalwart effort in joining in with the fun at the Mey Games. He became a great source of evening entertainment at the Castle and was often invited to join the QM in her lounge to sing and play his guitar. He was a songwriter and often used to entertain (once with the visiting Royal Family). He enjoyed singing Billy Connolly's 'Welly Song', one which went 'Ye cannae shove your granny off a bus' and one of his own favourites 'The Jeely Piece Song'. It is unreported whether anyone present understood the words to these songs, but the QM loved that sort of thing. It was reported quite recently that the record collection she kept at the Castle of Mey had included West Indian ska, local folk songs, Scottish reels and the musicals *Oklahoma!* and *The King and I*, along with recordings by comedians such as Tony Hancock and the Goons. So her taste in entertainment was wide.

As the time for HM to depart for Birkhall at Balmoral was getting close, we continued to have very good chats around the Policies. She let me know in various ways that she was happy with the way everything was going. During my time as her physician I'm pleased to say that she had very few problems on my watch, as it were; there was of course the occasion in 1982 before her visit to the Castle when she was admitted to King Edward VII Hospital to have a fish bone removed from her throat. She used to joke that it was the salmon's revenge!

With this event in mind I had written out a brief standing order for Sir Ralph that if she was ever taken seriously ill while at the Castle of Mey she should be flown to Aberdeen Royal Infirmary, where there were specialists that would look after her. She wasn't too sure about that, until she was told she would be taken by helicopter. That made it all right!

But what line could I take that would let me do research in the field of occupational medicine that HM might approve of? From now on, whether I liked it or not, I was associated with a member of the Royal Family, and everything I did must take that into account.

I mentioned to Sir Ralph that I was interested in the work and dangers facing the police officers of the Royal Protection Squad. The Queen Mother knew of my interest in their work. Although she never worried about her own safety, she was always very concerned about the welfare of her staff; she had been very upset when an officer was shot when a deranged attacker tried to kidnap the Princess Royal in Pall Mall in 1974.

I had occasion to discuss some issues with the Royal Protection Squad, who were a wonderful bunch. The squad came to my aid one day when my Range Rover had a puncture. Workmen had been repairing the castle roof, and the tyre had picked up a galvanised nail. The officers couldn't find the jack, so three of them just lifted it up while a fourth changed the wheel – most impressive! There was an occupational group I could use to start my occupational medicine research plans. That, I knew, would certainly meet with the QM's approval.

Sir Ralph jumped at this idea, and asked me if it would help if a post at Clarence House could be arranged. It might make a good base for my work, he said. It was thoughtful of him, but that would have been an honorary appointment, and I couldn't afford to move to London on that basis. He also suggested that if I wanted to go into private practice, he could arrange rooms in Harley Street, but I said it was now too late to start again and make my way in private practice.

I was effectively turning down the almost certain chance of a higher honour, but titles and honours really didn't bother me. My aims and goals were of much more importance to me, and with them the satisfaction that I knew would come from applying my knowledge and skills to the benefit of everyday workers. He was a little crestfallen, but fully understood the situation.

After my conversation with Sir Ralph I was greatly relieved that my plans were still on course, but I realised that everything I did from then I would have to do with the HM's approval in mind. How on earth would I know what she did or did not approve of? The Queen Mother never openly expressed approval for anything, and preferred to keep her thoughts and opinions very private. Often it was what she didn't say that gave us all a clue as to the way she was thinking.

Then Sir Ralph came up with a brilliant suggestion. He mentioned how many patronages the QM had – many were medically orientated and others were academic (she had recently given up the Chancellorship of London University, handing over to Princess Anne) and she had numerous honorary doctorates from the Medical Royal Colleges. It was clear where at least one of her interests lay, and I thought this could be a good starting point. The NHS was the largest employer in the country, and there was a huge variety of different occupational tasks with health implications and little or no research done into their occupational health problems. There were rumours going around that the NHS in England was setting up Occupational Health Services, and the Health Boards in Scotland were about ready to follow suit. This seemed to be just the outlet for my plans. I would now have to keep a lookout for any possible posts in Occupational Medicine.

It was a comfort to know that if I found a post of this nature I would still in a sense be a Physician (even more Extraordinary!) working 'On Her Majesty's Service'. I knew that HM always liked to know what was going on and would always be kept well informed.

It wasn't long before I heard that the Forth Valley Health Board NHS in the Central Scotland area was looking for a Consultant in Occupational Medicine to set up an Occupational Health Services Department and serve as its Director. This sounded as if it had great possibilities, and I went for it without a second thought.

The interview was demanding, with a larger panel than I expected. They were interested to hear my plans for future research, and these seemed to resonate with some of the members, one of whom I recognised as the Professor of Occupational Medicine at Aberdeen University.

After the interview I was taken to one side and informed that the position was mine. Kirstie was delighted when I told her my news, and I too was happy, for now I really was on my way to yet another new chapter in my life, with some fresh challenges and exciting work.

CHAPTER TEN

DRIVING FOR A HEALTHY WORKFORCE

In 1984 I resigned from my practice at Canisbay and we left the Health Board house. As a temporary measure we bought a house in Munlochy on the Black Isle, near Kirstie's parents, who were living in nearby Strathpeffer. I was provided with temporary living accommodation at one of the Health Board Hospitals and occupied the former Matron's suite, joining the family in Munlochy at weekends. This arrangement lasted for about a year, until we decided to look for a more permanent house closer to my work. We found the ideal place in Bridge of Allan near Stirling and moved there later that year.

My first priority as Director and Consultant involved setting up Occupational Health Service Units in each hospital and area within the Health Board. With the tremendous help of Barbara Healey, a senior Occupational

Health Nurse, and her nursing team, we set about the task, bringing new methods of clinical surveillance into the work of the centres. It was a formidable task, but we succeeded and eventually the service got up and running well.

With that completed, I set about doing some research into health problems in the NHS. This was a preliminary to applying the new approach to occupational health which I had brought with me from the RAF. I searched every sickness absence record I could find and held regular occupational health clinics to look for a pattern that might help me to make a start on the changes I wanted to bring about. I shadowed every occupational group within the hospital setting, learning as much as possible about the tasks involved in every area from the kitchens and laundries to the clinical areas. Even the offices of managers and administrators were not immune to my probings.

As I suspected, few if any studies like this had been carried out before, and the results clearly indicated that not only were there areas where quite serious health hazards existed but many of the employees who were off work with health problems came from areas where no obvious hazards had been suspected. Most interestingly, when I carried out a fuller investigation of their work tasks, I discovered that quite often their problems had started with a change of role, a change in the workplace or some additional factor that didn't appear to constitute a hazard in itself. It was back to the 'Whopperburger effect', where additions or changes could tip the employee out of the safety envelope. Now I knew exactly what I had to do.

The new techniques were beginning to look very promising. Most of the identified health problems at work could be rectified and the affected worker returned to duty by adopting fairly straightforward methods. These included modifying or removing the hazard, and we set up selective health surveillance programmes. We also introduced teaching and training where appropriate. My IAM and NASA approach to the problem was working. Human resources managers were delighted. No longer were they presented with the old solution of 'light duties only', which rarely or never existed, and sickness absence rates quite markedly declined.

Word spread quickly, and I was asked to take on an additional role as Director of Occupational Health for the CSA (Common Services Agency). This comprised a range of services for the NHS, including the blood transfusion service, prescription bureau and other less well-known bodies. Of greatest interest to me was that it included the whole of the Scottish Ambulance Service, and this was the one that presented the greatest challenge of all. I adopted the same approach and shadowed the ambulance crews on day and night shifts, observing every task they performed and measuring various physiological parameters as they carried it out. With the ambulance crews I attended every imaginable medical emergency, and some pretty horrific road traffic accidents and others. The pattern of health hazards facing the ambulance crews was very much the same as those in other NHS occupations, and the 'Protocol' helped to identify them and bring sickness absence under control.

One major health problem faced by ambulance staff was the stress and its effects brought about by harrowing incidents or accidents. Nowhere was this more apparent than the awful tragedy of Pan Am Flight 103, which crashed in Lockerbie in December 1988 with the loss of all aboard. It also brought about the deaths of some residents in the town itself. The response of the ambulance service to this dreadful catastrophe was immediate, and their pre-prepared disaster plan was put into action. The stress on the ambulance and other emergency services was enormous, due to the grim task of helping to collect bodies and bits of bodies from the accident scene; It was also made worse by the frustration that as there was nobody alive from the aircraft there was no opportunity for ambulance staff to apply the skills and assistance that they had been trained to provide.

This major incident added a new dimension to my research. I remained at Ambulance HQ during the first day of the incident, but the returning crews showed the classic signs and symptoms of post-traumatic stress, some of which lasted for days, sometimes weeks, and in a few cases for years. The staff of occupational health services from all over the country gave of their own time and joined forces with our staff to help deal with the situation. This was outside my field of experience, but with the help of psychiatrists and clinical psychologists I soon learned how best to deal with the condition.

The experience stood me in good stead for yet more harrowing and distressing events to come. The lessons we learned from the Pan Am 103 disaster unfortunately were needed again to cope with the aftermath of the tragedy that befell our nearby town of Dunblane. On the 13th March 1996, at the hands of a deranged gunman, sixteen little children and their teacher were mown down in the classroom of their primary school. The incident was of course indescribably distressing for the parents and relatives, but there was distress too for all those who were faced with such appalling scenes, including the police and ambulance crews. It took weeks of hard work in counselling to deal with the stress problems that resulted. It took that tragedy to point to ways we could prepare ambulance and police by teaching and making crews aware of the problems they might have to face in the course of their work. This was an adaptation of the approach used by NASA following some of their incidents and accidents.

On a lighter note, my passion for cars returned and I bought a Mazda MX3 sports car. The family were convinced I was entering a mid-life crisis, but it was great fun to drive and raising and lowering the hood was a doddle compared to the performance required with my previous sports models. The car was fun for two people, but useless for taking the family to school and a nightmare for carrying luggage in the boot. It was all you could do to pack a toothbrush in it for overnight stays. Still, it went like the wind, and with Japanese electronic wizardry the exhaust note was tuned to give a growl very reminiscent of the Aston Martin I once owned.

I was glad of the Mazda's speed and manoeuvrability when I was called out to an emergency at Glasgow Airport on Christmas Eve 1991. One of British Airways' planes had damaged its undercarriage on take-off from Sumburgh Airfield in Shetland and had radioed in an emergency alert, fearing that the undercarriage would not come down for landing. The emergency services were on standby at the airport and they were anxious for some reason to have an aviation-experienced doctor to examine the crew. I literally burned rubber to get from Bridge of Allan to the airport, but almost as I arrived the aircraft made a safe landing after a second attempt. Nobody was injured and I carried out my examination of the crew as asked to do so.

I heard no more about this incident, until later in the New Year a letter arrived at the house with the offer of two first-class tickets to Paris or New York. Kirstie and I opted for the latter, and flew out to the States in grand style, courtesy of British Airways. We landed in New York in a horrendous snowstorm. All the taxis and buses were full and there was a queue a mile long for any means of transport available into the centre of Manhattan. With a bit of luck we managed to secure a stretched limousine with enough room in it to hold a dance, complete with decanters of every kind of spirit you could imagine. At least it got us to our hotel, and we had a great few days exploring the delights of the city that never sleeps. We visited just about every tourist attraction and every major store and were exhausted by the end of the trip. At least it was a perk of the job and it came at a most opportune time.

Still the word was spreading, and more and more human resources departments were ringing up asking for occupational health advice and assistance with their sickness absence control. That was when I set up the OccuMedic Research Foundation. The original idea was to help students and field workers with their research projects, but we also managed to obtain funding to equip Stirling Ambulance Station with a small gymnasium and other sports equipment that would help to keep up their state of fitness. Most of all, the Foundation enabled me to extend occupational health advisory services to industry and businesses in the area, and boy did that bring some interesting results.

In a factory producing frozen chips for school and works

canteens, I came up against an unusual occupational hazard. Some of the workers complained that they couldn't lose weight because they were constantly breathing in fumes from the fat fryers used in the process. It took quite a bit of convincing that inhaling fat wasn't the cause of the problem and fat fumes did not constitute an occupational hazard.

I had a conscience however giving that advice, because on every visit to the factory I would be asked to taste samples of chips in the test laboratory. At ten o'clock in the morning that was inexcusable, and I paid the price by enlarging my waistline. So eating though not inhaling fat was perhaps an occupational hazard after all – for doctors!

My involvement with industry grew, and I was making visits to chemical plants, factories and other heavy industrial sites. In them all, the new method of investigating their health problems revealed hazards they hadn't spotted, and I was able to advise on steps to reduce their sickness absence. Studies of other occupations like lorry driving showed that in addition to the known risk of back pain from lifting heavy loads, the ergonomics of the lorry cab and the drivers' sitting posture also played a part. It was reminiscent of my studies into back pain in Hunter pilots back in the Bahrain days. Like that problem from the past, it was teaching and familiarisation training and other simple measures that brought the problem under control.

Perhaps it was when I got involved in investigating and advising local councils on occupational health that I unearthed the most extraordinary causes of sickness absence in their workforces. Part of my new protocol was to shadow employees doing every type of working task. I went out with the dustbin collectors and looked at what was involved in their work. I worked with employees in a sewage plant and studied every task that was going on there. Most of the workers in these areas were aware of the dangers in the workplace and of the care that must be taken to avoid chemical hazards and biological contamination, but few realised the nature of the material they were handling. This came to light when one worker spreading sewage in a landfill site dropped his sandwich on the ground, picked it up, rubbed it 'clean' on his sleeve and ate it! No worries, he thought, because it was treated sewage. But I discovered that by 'treatment' they meant squeezing raw sewage between rollers to remove water and create a more manageable sludge. It was still the same highly dangerous material as it was before.

That and other practices had to be put right, and I did so by setting up education talks for the workforce, greater health surveillance and provided protective equipment. In this way we helped to reduce health hazards and sickness absence fell.

Council-run activities like swimming pools and even libraries were throwing up all kinds of health hazards, and never a day went by when another occupation and another workforce were not calling for my services. It was hectic, but immensely satisfying. I just hoped that my involvement with some of these occupations hadn't reached the ears of the Queen Mother - but then I was her 'Extraordinary Physician' and I'm sure it would have greatly amused her.

It was about this time that my second son Willie began to take an interest in flying. At the first opportunity he took lessons at a flying club in Edinburgh. On his sixteenth birthday one of our friends, Captain Elliott Stenhouse, a Training Captain with British Airways, invited Willie and me to join him at the BA Simulator at Cranebank, near

Heathrow. Willie was thrilled to bits to be allowed to 'fly' in the left hand seat, and despite his age and inexperience he performed very well on a simulated flight from London Heathrow to Manchester. He was a complete natural, and I knew from that moment that he was destined to become an airline pilot.

This birthday present strengthened his interest in all things aviation, and he joined the Dunblane Air Cadets. He talked me into acting as the Reviewing Officer for the annual parade, but I had put on weight and my uniform, last used many years previously, was unbearably tight. Despite that, it was fun to see father and son both wearing RAF uniform. It was a moment I will always treasure.

Willie also persuaded me to renew my authorisation by the CAA to carry out annual and six-monthly medical examinations of airline, commercial and private fliers. Although it was an activity that didn't contribute anything much to my research work in Occupational or Aviation Medicine, it was a welcome diversion from the busy working life I was leading.

Dr Iain Symington, my opposite number in the Greater Glasgow Health Board, also persuaded me to join him in carrying out medical examinations on behalf of the DVLA. To begin with the examinations were to assess the fitness of drivers who were suffering from various medical conditions or recovering from surgery that might affect their ability to drive. That made use of our clinical and ergonomic skills, and it was greatly satisfying to be able to advise on modifications to a vehicle that would allow these people to return to driving. Sometimes it was quite a difficult decision when it stopped someone from driving and prevented them from getting about, but it just had to be done as part of the job.

On one occasion, I was approached by the Matron of a nursing home and asked to persuade a very elderly lady in her care to give up her driving licence. Technically she was fit enough to continue to hold one, but when I learned that she had purchased a new extremely powerful Kawasaki motorcycle and saw no reason why she couldn't ride it, I shared Matron's concern. I finally persuaded her that it was time to hang up her riding leathers, and she reluctantly agreed – much to everybody's relief.

Then the emphasis of the work changed, and we became swamped with the examination of drivers who had been disqualified for drink-driving offences. The assessment of their fitness or otherwise to hold a driving licence was made from blood samples we took at the clinic, and the decision was based entirely on the results of laboratory tests that we sent to the DVLA in Swansea.

I got weary of the failure to use any of my clinical or physiological skills in the decision-making process. The last straw came when the emphasis yet again changed to assessing drivers trying to renew their licence after a drug-driving conviction. I had to put up with verbal, and occasional, physical abuse from applicants who were high on drugs, and in the end I could take no more, and gave up these clinics once and for all.

I was still very much aware that I had not had time to address a problem which I knew to be dear to the heart of the Queen Mother - the dangers to which officers of the Royal Protection Squad and other police officers are exposed. I remembered the offer which Sir Ralph Anstruther had made when we discussed my future career pathway. He had suggested that I might find it useful to set up a base in London so that I would have ready access to the Metropolitan Police who made up the Protection Squad. To assess the feasibility of doing this and through the good offices of Clarence House, I managed to get rooms in Harley Street, as Sir Ralph had suggested. For two or three months I commuted on a weekly basis to London, but I found the travelling just too exhausting on top of all my other commitments. By the time my plane had got into Heathrow and I had struggled through the heavy traffic, the commissionaire on the door had gone for lunch, the lift was not available and the climb up several flights of stairs to my consulting room on the top floor left me with little time or energy to do any worthwhile research work. I realised it just wasn't going to work, and I reluctantly gave up the idea as wholly impractical.

The exercise had however given me the opportunity to sail up river on a Thames water taxi to visit my eldest son Russell, who had a flat in Cascades in the Docklands. This was shades of the Sharps of two centuries before, who as I mentioned in Chapter 2 loved nothing more than to go for musical cruises on the same river. It also fulfilled a rather silly ambition of mine to have my name on a brass plate in Harley Street - always a sign among consultant colleagues that you had finally arrived!

Through the nineties, snippets of news about the Queen Mother's deteriorating state of health began to filter through, and this caused me some anxiety. She was getting on in years - in fact she was heading for her centenary in 2000 - and I realised that unless I could find some way of investigating the health at work problems of the Royal Protection Squad, as I had promised to do, it might be too late. I was in a dilemma. I had so many balls in the air with my work in Scotland that I couldn't see any hope of getting any kind of research programme off the ground.

Then something of a minor miracle happened which changed all that. I was asked to meet with the Chief Inspector and his instructor staff at the Traffic Training Division of the Scottish Police College at Tulliallan Castle in Fife. There they explained that they had a serious and very worrying problem. There was a high incidence of road traffic accidents involving police vehicles. The puzzle was that many of these included highly-trained police drivers, and there was mounting concern among the Association of Chief Police Officers in England and their Scottish equivalent. They wondered if I could possibly investigate the problem.

Of course, I jumped at the chance of looking into the matter. Here was my opening into work on the health hazards of operational police driving, which of course would include the Royal Protection Squad. Perfect! I wasted no time in setting up my investigation.

With the co-operation of local police forces, I used the same approach I had used in every other workplace investigation. I joined the drivers of police traffic vehicles on every shift I could and shadowed them in every task they performed. These sometimes included night drives. We attended some horrific incidents and road traffic accidents, often meeting the ambulance crews I had worked with in a previous project. All these attendances involved highly-skilled driving, usually at speed and frequently in high-density traffic. I devised techniques for measuring a driver's vigilance throughout every phase of the drive and gathered stacks of results of physiological parameters throughout.

Analysis of the results showed that there were several previously unrecognised factors associated with this type of operational driving which could affect the skill of the driver, compromise his efficiency and safety and lead to accidents. The new protocol had worked like a dream again, and I was able to build up a profile of operational police driving and define a 'safety envelope' for each and every task.

The next phase was to make a few adjustments to police operational procedures which did not materially interfere with the task they were required to do. I returned to training, my old friend, and produced two videos to familiarise drivers with the hazards they faced. I also gave advice on ways of minimising the effects. I gave lectures on the subject to advanced courses, attending the College, and with the encouragement and assistance of Chief Inspector Andrew Bright and the Commandant at the time, Hugh Watson, I wrote a textbook called *Human Aspects of Police Driving*. At my request, all royalties from this publication went to Scottish Road Safety.

I was invited to attend the National Police Driving Schools Conference, where the Chairman directed that the book should become required reading for every police driving school throughout the country. I hadn't expected this to happen, nor was I really prepared for the lectures, demonstrations and presentations that flowed from it. I think I managed to visit every police training establishment in the country, including the Police Training College at Hendon. Here they gave me a brief introduction to Royal and VIP escort driving, and I could now understand the concerns of the Queen Mother.

I was invited to speak at many conferences and meetings,

including the Blue Light Users' Group, which included members of all the emergency services. I welcomed them all as a means of spreading the word.

Interest in my new experimental approach and protocol began to spread, and I was awarded a Fellowship of the Faculty of Occupational Medicine with a very nice citation from the President of the Royal College of Physicians himself (he was later to become Physician to HM the Queen). There followed other academic awards, including Fellowship of the Royal College of Physicians and Surgeons, Glasgow. I had quite a conscience accepting this, as it was awarded without examination, and I felt for all the poor aspiring clinicians who had to take very stiff examinations to gain the Membership, far less the Fellowship.

At this time my academic work was piling up, and I was heavily involved in lecturing to students from the Department of Community Medicine at Glasgow. Then came the rather odd situation when I was invited to give the annual lecture on Aviation Physiology at Glasgow University as a Visiting Professor. It felt strange to be standing in front of students in this old lecture theatre. It seemed smaller than in my student days, but then everything seems that way as you get older. It was of course at Glasgow University where Bill Stewart had sparked my interest in aviation medicine off many years before when he had been Commandant of IAM, and it was where I had had my baptism of fire as a junior lecturer. I fully expected the ball bearings to come down the steps, followed by a paper aeroplane on fire, as in the old days, but they didn't come and it turned out to be an enjoyable and valuable experience to meet up-and-coming doctors who were interested in aviation and occupational medicine. I was so pleased that young people were considering these unusual and perhaps extraordinary career pathways.

Interest in the textbook and my investigation methods spread abroad. First the Swedish police invited me to give a lecture to almost their entire force in a huge hall in the city of Gothenburg. It was not helped by the fact that of course I couldn't speak a word of Swedish, although the senior police officers who invited me were absolutely insistent that everyone understood English. I have no idea whether the audience gained much from my talk, but the welcome and hospitality were overwhelming.

After the lecture I was taken out to the old Volvo car proving track some miles out of the City. There they demonstrated their training procedures for police and other emergency services drivers and allowed me to experience these in a police car which cleverly converted to a skid training vehicle. It was just as well the large traffic cone dressed up as a little girl wasn't real, as I hit 'her' on several occasions during my very amateur efforts to control a skidding vehicle. I was learning fast.

A trip in a police helicopter to view the dense traffic conditions on the road system leading into and out of the City added to my experiences. The kind invitation by the pilot to take the controls added to my own stress levels, but these were nothing compared to the stress of the next part of my visit, which involved a demonstration of high speed manoeuvring through very dense traffic on the highway. I just hoped they had understood some of content of the lecture and might get the chance to read my book.

A visit from some very senior police officers from the

People's Democratic Republic of China to the College at Tulliallan caused a degree of confusion. They had asked for the textbook to be written in Chinese, and with the help of a translation service in London we were able to print off enough pre-publication copies to show them during their visit. Panic set in when the translator from the Chinese Embassy in London asked whether the final edition would be in Mandarin or Cantonese. At enormous expense to the College we were prepared to print hundreds of copies, half in Mandarin and the other in Cantonese. It was only much later that we discovered that the difference between the two was mainly one of dialect, and made little difference to the printed word. Thank goodness, as it would have depleted Scottish Police funds in a big way.

The lecture I gave to the group was a protracted affair. Every sentence had to be translated into Chinese, and when thankfully I got to the end and offered as usual to answer any questions, I was met by stony silence. I was sure they hadn't understood a single word and that it had all been a waste of time and effort, but they had taken it all in. Much of it had been captured on personal recorders or on cameras thrust in my face at regular times during the talk.

I later discovered that in Chinese culture, to have asked a question would imply that they hadn't understood the content, and that would have been very rude and discourteous. We live and learn.

We also had a very interesting and fruitful visit from the United States Federal Law Enforcement Agency. They had a massive training establishment in Glynn County in Georgia, and were anxious for me to join their training team on a sabbatical as what they referred to as a Distinguished Visiting

Professor. What excited me about this offer was that they hoped to build up a television centre which would transmit training programmes to outlying police units. This was exactly what I wanted to do, and it promised to let me apply everything I had learned from RAF AMTC and my time with ITN. I accepted the offer immediately and was looking forward eagerly to the experience. As it turned out the Agency, like us, had their funding problems, and Congress cancelled the project, so that was an end to my involvement.

I then retired from my NHS post as Consultant and Director of Occupational Health Services. This gave me the opportunity to concentrate on work with the Scottish Police College, and the scope of my research extended to other areas of police work. I had now almost reached my goal, and was looking towards retirement at long last and the rare opportunity to take things easy for a change.

With the new millennium, which we managed to see in as a family, I tried to wind down my work and keep on a few projects that interested me. In 2000 I was invited to attend a dinner at the Police College on the 17th April, and Kirstie and I attended the function with no knowledge of what was in store. At the end of the dinner the Commandant announced that I was to receive a unique award, HRH Prince Michael of Kent's Special Award for Contribution to Road Safety. I was amazed to receive such an honour, which was the best 65th Birthday and retirement present I could have been given.

It was two days later that tragedy struck our family.

On the 19th of April we were expecting Willie home, because he had said he was coming up to have his car serviced in Stirling. He never turned up, and when I phoned him, there was no answer. Our daughter Melanie called, with the same result. We went to bed; perhaps he would turn up in the morning. It was Easter and his airline would be busy. Perhaps he had been called out to stand in for another first officer unable to fly. But at 4 am there came a knock on the door and I opened it to reveal a young policeman.

'Dr Sharp?' he said. I confirmed I was. 'May I suggest that you sit down please sir?' he said.

I knew immediately that something was terribly wrong. The officer explained. It turned out that Willie had died from a cerebral haemorrhage as a result of a berry aneurysm, a ballooning of a brain artery bursting.

It was impossible to believe; it still is. Willie was a big, strong fit chap who had never had a day's illness and he was only 24 years old, so talented and with all his life and his career ahead of him. We could only console ourselves with the thought that at least it hadn't happened when he had been flying.

The loss of Willie took a huge chunk out of all our lives. You never get over such a loss; you can only try to learn to live with it. Christmas and family occasions can be very difficult, as we can never put the empty seat at table out of our minds. But there were other members of the family to think about, and Kirstie and I just had to get on with life.

In 2005 Kirstie took part in the London Marathon in memory of Willie. She collected quite a nice sum of money for the charity the Brain and Spine Foundation, and later collected her medal as she crossed the finishing line after an amazing effort for someone who was untrained and had no track record, if you'll forgive the pun, as an athlete. Russell, Melanie and I were there in London to support her during the event, and we were all extremely proud of her for managing to complete the course.

I began to shed most of my work and decided to take full retirement. I had little appetite for my work after our sad loss, but I kept on the Civil Aviation Authority medicals because I knew this was what Willie would have wanted me to do. The contact with his old airline chums who visited the house for their medicals helped Kirstie and me to cope with our loss, and it kept me in touch with what was going on in the airline industry.

In May of 2001, a nondescript brown envelope arrived by post at our house in Bridge of Allan. It was the run up to the General Election and we were daily being deluged with election bumf which came in with every post. When I saw the address of origin was 10 Downing Street I assumed it was another leaflet urging me to vote in favour of one party or the other. My first inclination was to tear it up and throw it into the waste paper basket along with all the others.

Just as well I didn't. It was a letter to inform me that the Prime Minister had it mind on the occasion of the forthcoming list of Birthday Honours to submit my name to the Queen with recommendation for appointment as a Member of the Most Excellent Order of the British Empire (MBE).

I almost collapsed on the floor, and when I recovered from the shock I wondered how this had come about. I had my suspicions, but recipients are never told anything about these matters. I did however learn unofficially that it was for my contribution to police driver training, so perhaps my suspicions were correct!

When the big day arrived for the investiture, Kirstie, Melanie and Alastair were allocated places in the Ballroom at Buckingham Palace to watch the ceremony. It was awe inspiring, though without too much pomp and circumstance, and when I went up to the dais to receive my medal from HRH Prince Charles my legs turned to jelly. The Prince seemed to know a lot about my work, and mentioned the Royal Protection Squad in the conversation. He must have been well briefed, as there was no mention of that part of my work in the citation.

As the four of us walked out into the sunshine of the Mall, I looked back at the dazzling edifice of Buckingham Palace. It had been a wonderful and magical day, the crowning glory of a career that had taken me on a long and at times tortuous pathway to my goal, and to this previously undreamed-of honour. As an ordinary physician who had benefited from some extraordinary luck (and perhaps a little hard work), I could not have asked for a more wonderful ending.

EPILOGUE

Not long after the investiture we bought a new house in Fortrose, with spectacular views across the Black Isle and over to the Moray Firth. Although I had kept on with my CAA clinics with pilots coming to the house for medicals, much of my time was now my own. I occupied myself with landscaping the rocky, steeply-sloping field which eventually became our garden, and generally doing odd jobs and helping Kirstie around the house.

I still felt the urge to keep up to date with what was going on in the field of civil aviation, and one day I attended a meeting of CAA Authorised Medical Examiners. During the coffee break I found myself talking to a young doctor who told me that he was hoping to take the Diploma in Occupational Medicine. He explained that it had become *the* speciality to be in, and was now up there beside the other specialists like surgeons and physicians. 'What I like about it is that it combines the skill of a doctor with science and even engineering, and there's great scope for research,' he told me.

He went on to describe some of the techniques that were being used. He didn't know me from Adam, so he had no idea that I had introduced many of them myself.

'Most of the research work in the specialty is based on aviation medicine, you know, and I think it won't be long before there could be a manned spaceflight to Mars' he said.

'That should be interesting', I replied. 'I would love to be involved in that somehow when it happens.'

I was happy to hear that the younger generation of doctors looked on aviation and space medicine as a part of occupational medicine. That was the best reward I could have hoped for, and it gave me great hope for the future. But beyond that, the encounter with that doctor got me thinking. I started to wonder about the problems of manned interplanetary spaceflight. It all seemed feasible enough to me. I knew that most of the physiological challenges had been thoroughly studied and overcome in various ways. I felt sure we would be seeing men on Mars in no time.

Pondering the matter some time later over a cup of coffee, I opened the kitchen door to the sunshine and wandered down to the end of our garden, where our gardener, Mike Wood, was hard at work.

'Morning, Mike' I greeted him.

'Morning', he said, with his usual cheerful grin. 'Heard on the news this morning that they might be flying men to Mars in the next few years.'

'Yes, I heard that too' I replied. 'And it's beginning to look as if it is really quite possible.'

'I wouldn't like to be stuck in a spacecraft' said Mike. 'It would give me cabin fever.'

'Cabin fever?' I repeated.

'Yes, I used to get it as a lad and I still do when it's nasty weather and I can't get out of the house. The worst part about it is that the longer it goes on the worse it gets. It can drive you crazy.'

I froze on the spot. With that casual remark, Mike had put his finger on a crucial flaw in the preparations for the Mars mission. Of course - it wasn't the physiological problems but the psychological ones that were the real challenge. They could so easily put the kybosh on the whole venture or at least delay it until the 2020s or later.

But what had stopped me dead in my tracks was the last part of Mike's observation, where he had observed 'it gets worse with time'. This change with time could seriously alter all previously calculated 'safety operating envelopes' for long-term space travel. We would need to know very much more about the way psychological problems like 'cabin fever' develop and change with time into the mission. We know from previous spaceflights that an overwhelming sense of isolation and its associated symptoms appear to set in at about the halfway stage of the mission. And we know from the Russian-led experiment confining people to a simulated spacecraft cabin for over 500 days that debilitating effects (anxiety, loneliness, depression, irritability and insomnia) can seriously compromise the safety of the mission. But how do these symptoms change with time, and how do they interact with other factors in the spaceflight? These are the questions that must be answered before we can calculate 'safety envelopes' for interplanetary travel.

'You know Mike, you've hit the nail on the head' I said. 'And what's more, you've just rekindled an old interest of mine in long-term space travel. Cabin fever is just the problem I'm going to start with. It will be a challenge to see what on Earth we can do about that. Or on Mars, I should say.'

As I walked briskly back up to the house, I remembered Sir James Black's advice to me all those years ago at the start of my career: 'Never let your last goal be your last achievement' he had wisely told me. Now I knew there was still some exciting work for me to do. I was going to start by working out a brand new 'flight profile' and define a new 'safety envelope' for future Mars missions.

Now, where had I left those original papers and calculations?